THE
DREAMING
PATH

THE DREAMING PATH

INDIGENOUS WISDOM,
MEDITATIONS, AND EXERCISES
TO LIVE OUR BEST STORIES

Paul Callaghan *with* **Uncle Paul Gordon**

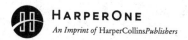
HarperOne
An Imprint of HarperCollins*Publishers*

While this book is intended as a general information resource and all care has been taken in compiling the contents, it does not take account of individual circumstances and is not in any way intended as a substitute for professional medical or psychological advice, diagnosis, or treatment. It is essential that you always seek advice from a qualified health professional if you suspect you have a health problem. The author and publisher disclaim any liability in connection with the use of or reliance on the information contained in this book.

The information in this book is published in good faith and for general information purposes only. Although the author and publisher believe at the time of going to press that the information is correct, they do not assume and hereby disclaim any liability to any party for any loss, damage, or disruption caused by errors or omissions, whether they result from negligence, accident, or any other cause.

Some passages in this book include knowledge and cultural expressions of Aboriginal and Torres Strait Islander peoples. This knowledge comes from Country and its people and has been handed down through the generations. It is Indigenous Cultural and Intellectual Property (ICIP) that belongs communally to First Peoples, who continue to practice their culture. First Peoples have cultural protocols about how their ICIP can be shared and used, and the unauthorized use, adaptation, and publication of ICIP without the free prior informed consent of First Peoples is a breach of ICIP protocols.

Originally published in Australia in 2022 by Pantera Press Pty Limited.

FIRST HARPERCOLLINS PAPERBACK PUBLISHED IN 2024

Design adapted by Terry McGrath from the Australian edition designed by Pantera Press Pty Limited.

Library of Congress Cataloging-in-Publication Data is available upon request.

ISBN 978-0-06-332127-4

24 25 26 27 28 LBC 5 4 3 2 1

To those who are ready to shed their
cloak of gray and dance in color.

To my wife, Alison, who has taught me so many things.

To those who have come before me.
I hope I have honored your footsteps.

Contents

The Message

The big sky slumbered in its enormity. The stars looked down on the ancient sands with infinite memories of what had been. The orange of small flames pierced the darkness. By the firelight I sat, hypnotized by the profound stillness. The crackle and fizz of the embers amplified the quiet as wisps of smoke began to take shape. The Old Spirit looked at me with eyes of wisdom, love, and sadness.

Why are you all so busy but doing so little? Why do you try so hard to get things you don't really need? Why do you see happiness as such a hard thing to achieve? Why can't you be content with what you have been given? What you really need is all around you, but you don't see it.

You have all lost your way. You have forgotten who you are.

You are not living your truth.

You still have time to remember. You need to remember. You need to reconnect. If you don't remember, if you don't reconnect, you will have failed us, and things that are important will be gone . . . we will be gone . . . everything will be gone . . . and lost . . . forever.

Preface

We, the authors of this book, pay our respects to and acknowledge all Indigenous peoples of this earth, past, present, and future.

As Aboriginal people from the lands now called Australia, we honor the many traditional Aboriginal Nations within Australia. We pay our respects to our Aboriginal Elders across Australia and acknowledge their wisdom and guidance. We also acknowledge the ancestral animals that traveled Country long before we came to be, creating the rivers, mountains, and other landscapes before resting in the land itself. There are sacred places of respect and remembrance throughout Australia that connect us all.

We have written this book with love and with a desire to share appropriate knowledge with all who will listen. We do this with the belief that Indigenous cultures around the globe, including Australian Aboriginal culture, have the power to provide significant healing to the world.

Special care has been taken to ensure that the Old People would consider the knowledge we share appropriate to share with the general public. We respect the special nature of Aboriginal cultural and spiritual knowledge and have gone to great lengths to ensure we do not disclose any information that might be considered inappropriate.

We acknowledge we can only speak from our perspective and cannot speak on behalf of any other Aboriginal peoples or groups. Any resemblance in information contained in this book to that of other Aboriginal Nations or communities is unintentional but somewhat unavoidable, given the relationships that have been sustained and stories that have been shared across this vast land since the beginning.

It is our hope that if we share our knowledge, thoughts, and experiences, the reader will be inspired to seek cultural knowledge, insight, and context locally from the Elders and knowledge owners of the many Indigenous Nations that have cared for Country and continue to care for Country across the world. The stories we share have been created to demonstrate the beauty and wisdom of our culture. Most are new, but some are our interpretation of old stories that have been passed on to us. We share these old stories as a sign of respect for those who have shared this wisdom with us.

—Paul Callaghan and Uncle Paul Gordon

Being Aboriginal is not the color of your skin but your connection and responsibility to Country and all things in nature. It is about your connection to trees, fish, birds, rivers, rocks, and stars. It isn't about how you look. It isn't even about your bloodlines. It is about something unseen, deep inside you.

—UNCLE PAUL GORDON

THE
DREAMING
PATH

Introduction

In Aboriginal spirituality, everything is conceived . . . all things become pregnant . . . trees, plants, insects, birds, fish, reptiles, mammals, rocks . . . and eventually give birth.

The birth of this book is the result of 60,000 years of gestation. It contains knowledge and story that have been passed on for more than 1,800 generations.

Some people might be thinking, So? What use would a book based on a different culture from a different world be to me as I try to balance the demands of work, paying the bills, and doing my best to be a good person?

To answer that question, I would like to ask you to let go of the present for just a moment.

I would like to ask you to imagine a world with no war . . . no crime . . . no homelessness . . . no hunger . . . and no poverty. A world where every person has all they need to live a long life of fulfillment and well-being. A world with many languages but where there is no word for "hate" because "hate" does not exist.

You can let go of imagining now and come back to the present.

Do you think the kind of world described above can really exist? Most people would say no. They would say that history shows us human beings, by nature, do inhuman things to each other. They would say that over many thousands of years we have demonstrated we are incapable of uniting in a loving and caring way.

I disagree. The utopia described above was how Aboriginal people lived for a very, very long time. Yes, there were instances of disagreement and anger, but as you read this book you will gain an understanding of the systems, rules, and obligations in traditional Aboriginal society that created a way of life the analytical mind finds hard to accept. The traditional Aboriginal world functioned in a different time, but I am going to show you how traditional values, ways of thinking, and practices are just as applicable now. Perhaps even more so.

The world today has many things that give us joy and inspiration. Sunsets and sunrises, rainbows, snow-covered mountains, a child's laughter, hot water, chocolate, and the smell of coffee are things that lift my spirits and immerse me in bliss for a moment or two. And the ability to connect with a loved one who lives far away by phone, video link, plane, or vehicle is a remarkable testimony to the benefits of scientific and technological advancement.

But as I reflect on everything around me, although I know everyone is trying their hardest to do their best, I see too many faces lined with anxiety and stress. I see too few faces that emanate inner peace or contentment. I see too many people who appear to be going around in circles.

For me, the world is a magical place where I can see, hear, touch, taste, and smell an abundance of treasures, even when I am having one of those tough days when nothing seems to go right.

I haven't always had this outlook. Once upon a time, mine was one of those faces etched with determination but lacking in luster.

For more than sixty years I have been privileged to walk this earth. I have been through many of the peaks and troughs of life that we all must face. Like most people my age, I have navigated family grief, personal illness, paying bills, raising a family, and pursuing a career while also trying to be a good son, brother, husband, father, friend, and colleague.

My navigation process Before Culture was much more difficult than Post-Culture. The many things Aboriginal culture has given me have enabled me to achieve a state of mind, body, and spirit wellness I never thought possible. This book provides numerous insights and messages that can help you do the same.

The privilege of writing this book with Paul Gordon (Uncle Paul), a person of considerable insight, generosity, and patience (much needed with a protégé like me), is something I could not possibly have imagined years ago when I looked into the mirror. This book will reawaken your appreciation of the power of story.

The sharing of story is a cornerstone of Aboriginal culture. Story gives us time to slow down. Story connects us. Story teaches us.

But . . . before Uncle Paul and I share with you the wisdom of the ancient ones, I would like to share with you the story of how I was given access to the knowledge of the world's oldest living culture. Was it an accident or was it destiny? You can make up your own mind as you read on. What I do know is that this learning changed my life—it possibly saved my life. It is knowledge that is so simple to understand and yet so profound in its application. And it is here for all of us to consider, embrace, and live, if we are ready for the responsibilities that come with it. When I was thirty-four years old, I was the great Western success story. I had three degrees, two jobs, three kids, two cars, a house, and was married to the love of my life. I was living the dream. Despite all of this, on the day of my thirty-fifth birthday I sat on some steps at my workplace and cried. The tears continued for many months. Darkness, anxiety, and fear saturated my soul. The happy-go-lucky, always busy, indestructible mask of bravado I had worn for so long cracked and then fell apart, leaving me feeling naked, vulnerable, and exposed.

The psychiatrist diagnosed me with major depression and anxiety disorder. I went and researched these sinister words, "... and the darkness went several shades darker." Reading about depression made me more depressed. I was told there was no cure and that my condition would be a permanent one I could learn to manage at best.

One day I sat by the water's edge thinking, *This is the moment to end it.* The thought of ending my life was a compelling one. I saw it as the best way to free my family from the burden of having to care for someone with a permanent mental illness. But then a random thought came to me that betrayed my plan: *Maybe I don't need to believe the labels. Maybe I can learn from this experience and prove the experts wrong.*

And so started the process of healing. When I started to look deep inside, I found there were missing pieces ... undefined and intangible ... dark spaces in my spirit that moved and hid whenever my gaze turned toward them. I was searching for personal meaning: something to fill a void that no amount of career, monetary, or other external success could fill.

I read books. Lots of books. Books on the various world spiritualities. Self-help books. Books on mental health. Books on brain physiology. Books on happiness. Books on depression.

I tapped into other people—alternative healers, psychologists, and psychiatrists, and in men's groups and meditation groups. I practiced yoga, exercised a lot, created artworks, enjoyed my guitar, and learned all sorts of ways to breathe.

The missing pieces were slowly becoming more defined when something serendipitous happened. I was invited to go bush and learn about my culture.

This invitation had come as a major surprise. I had always felt proud of my Aboriginal heritage but had been told that traditional culture was long gone. Now here I was, in the bush, about to be given my first insight into our old ways.

The first thing I was shown was the smoking ceremony, and the importance of smoking yourself before going onto a site was explained. As I listened, a calmness and inner joy that I had never felt before cradled me. With the smell of smoke and gum leaves lingering in my nostrils, I was escorted through the post-sunset murkiness to a sheer, plain-looking bed of rock. I followed in a somber march of respect, wanting to show my thankfulness for what I was about to receive.

My teacher pointed to a place for me to stand and then bathed the rock in front of me with light. Suddenly, before me was a figure that had lain in stone for tens of thousands of years.

Words cannot describe how privileged I felt when my teacher shared the story of the engraving with me. As I listened, the analyst part of my brain marveled at how many generations of Aboriginal people had been to this very place and stood where I now stood. The creative part of my brain admired the beauty of the story I was being told, and the philosopher part of my brain was awestruck by the insight it contained. My heart felt like it would burst as my lifelong thirst for cultural knowledge was now being quenched.

In a world far beyond the constraints of the brain, my spirit awoke and danced as I connected to a place beyond that which is imaginable. It was a place of safety and it was a place of peace. I was infused by profound wisdom and felt unconditional, infinite love. I liked this place.

Over the next twelve months or so I went bush every week, sometimes twice a week. During this time, I learned about our creation and I learned about our Creator. I learned about Mother Earth, our relationship with everything that exists on the earth and in the sky, and I learned about the importance of being loving, respectful, and humble in all that I do. Most of all, I learned about myself. After many years of being lost in depression, I was finally able to begin to slowly replace my world of darkness and negativity with one of color, light, and hope through the healing and insight that culture gave me.

In this, my burray phase of learning (burray is a traditional word for "child" in the Gathang language), I was told of a man named Uncle Paul Gordon. Whenever his name was mentioned, it was done so with extreme reverence, which challenged my ego. In my mind, I was somewhat skeptical of the guru-like status given to this person.

When I first met Uncle Paul, the aloof cynicism I had affected so readily for so long evaporated the instant I felt his presence.

Although he was quiet and unassuming in every aspect of his demeanor, there was something about him that commanded respect. I immediately regretted my arrogance and judgment as I recognized a person who honored and walked his truth.

That was more than twenty years ago now. The road of recovery was a long one, potholed with disappointments, setbacks, and an underlying, pervasive fear that I would never get back to the old me. Upon reflection, and with much gratitude, I can say that my anxiety was misplaced. My journey of contemplation, healing, and growth enabled me to become the real me . . . a better me. The cornerstone of this profound, life-changing transformation was meeting Uncle Paul.

Over the time I have known Uncle Paul, he has transitioned from a figure I questioned, to a figure I feared, to a revered teacher, to an important mentor, to a trusted friend, to a treasured best friend. And although I have consumed only a small morsel of the banquet of cultural learning that he has shown me, I will be forever grateful for the nourishment it provides.

Uncle Paul is much farther along the path of learning than myself, of course, but by his own admission, even he is nowhere near the end.

His profound and life-changing knowledge is provided throughout this book. To ensure authenticity of context and meaning, whenever Uncle Paul's thoughts are shared, I have quoted him directly in the different font below. Here is the first passage:

I am a Ngemba man from northwestern New South Wales, born of Gurulgilu Country, meaning I belong to the stones. In our story, stones are born, stones have babies, stones grow, stones have spirit, and stones die like all things do. My people are stone people. We come from the rocks.

Over my life I have spent a lot of time working with Aboriginal communities creating organizations that can help our people achieve improved well-being. I have also spent much of my life traveling Country and sitting in natural landscapes with Old Men across Australia, doing cultural activities that reconnect Lore Men and the old stories so we can take better care of each other and Mother Earth. If we care for the Mother, she will always give us all that we need.

Ideally, we would love to share our thoughts with you face-to-face walking Country and sitting in a circle around a fire. Who knows? One day, that might happen. In the meantime, this book is our way of taking you bush. It gives you the chance to listen to what we might say if you were with us in person as well as the chance to reflect on what has been shared with you as if you were sitting around the fire with us.

Uncle Paul's thoughts are based on what he has been given by the Old People plus his observations of what surrounds him. When I listen to him, I still have a tendency to become a child, mesmerized by newfound ways of seeing the world and how I can better connect with it.

To help others access the wisdom of our ancestors, I explore and add to Uncle Paul's comments and thoughts, viewing them through lenses including:

- my cultural learning,
- my Western world learning,

- my lived experience,
- relevant Western research, and
- relevant Western theory and practice.

When I spoke at an international Indigenous healing confer-ence near San Francisco in 2017, a fellow delegate described me as a walker of many worlds. I quite liked that description.

The intent of the book is to provide you with Aboriginal cul-tural insights and points of reflection that you can use to:

- build your capacity to do things that will generate personal growth, greater meaning, and increased contentment in your daily life (inward perspective); and
- make your street, your community, your nation, and the world a better place for current and future generations (outward perspective).

Both perspectives are equally important.

To achieve our intent, we will be focusing a great deal on the Lore, from an English word that can be considered to mean the traditional knowledge passed on from generation to generation (through song, story, sites, and dance) that guides all aspects of our life. The traditional wording that captures the concept of the Lore differs across the continent, as can interpretations of its meaning; however, in essence, the Lore states we all have a responsibility to care for our place and all things in our place.

A Lore Man's role is also to share appropriate knowledge from the Lore with those who live on this land (regardless of where they might have been born) and want to learn to love and care for this country as much as Aboriginal people do. The relationship between the well-being of Country and our own well-being is symbiotic. If we fail to care for Country, the Mother's well-being will begin to suffer and, eventually, so will ours.

In addition to building a loving relationship with the land, our well-being is also dependent on our ability to build meaningful relationships with each other. A review of world history suggests that achieving this on a global scale has not been easy, to say the least. Recent news broadcasts involving items such as Black Lives Matter protests, wars, terrorism events, and disagreements between governments on global issues such as the climate crisis, poverty, religious practice, and trade indicate we have many obstacles to overcome.

In traditional Aboriginal society, this was not the case. The highly sophisticated governance, education, and kinship systems practiced across more than five hundred Aboriginal Nations ensured continuous connectivity through a platform of spiritual and familial unity that enabled diversity and difference to be understood, acknowledged, respected, and accepted. This state of being explains why there can be several Dreamtime stories about the same event.

Even though some of the stories are different, they have similar themes. Some of these stories with similar themes travel right across Australia and connect people together. In the old way, new stories are taken on board as long as these new stories don't take away from the old stories. Old and new stories can sit together and complement each other as long as the new stories value nature, all things in nature and our place. The stories in this book are some of many that can connect with many other stories throughout Australia and help connect us across the world.

Just as the stories in this book can connect us, so too can the insights provided by other spiritualities from around the world. *The Dreaming Path* does not intend to replace or position itself above any of these sources of inspiration and guidance. It aims to be a vehicle of transformation that sits alongside them.

There isn't one succinct method to guarantee a life of well-being and contentment, and we do not pretend this book has all the answers. It does, however, provide perspectives and ways of thinking that you could apply in some aspects of your life.

If people disagree with any of the views we express, we accept that difference of opinion with humility and grace. Diversity of opinion is, in itself, a marvelous opportunity for mutual exploration, conversation, learning, and growth. The world has lots of stories and lots of answers. It is our belief that there doesn't have to be one opinion, one truth, or one way of doing things.

In this journey of life, all you really have is your story. As the author of your story, it is important to reflect on everything you are told in order for you to decide what is relevant in your life and how you want your story to read. Too often, and sometimes without us even knowing it, we hand over authorship of our story to others and then wonder why we feel lost.

By owning your story, by analyzing what fits and what doesn't fit with it, and by coupling this with trust in your intuitive self, you will find it much easier to navigate the journey we call life in a way that is purposeful, inspired, authentic, and meaningful.

Each one of us is conceived and born for a purpose. Each one of us has a journey, a path we are meant to follow. There might be many potholes, barriers, and detours on the road ahead, but even these can become wonderful experiences and opportunities if we have the right attitude. Some of these perceived hurdles might seem insurmountable, but with insight, faith, belief, and effort, the amazing is within reach for us all. In fact, the amazing is already within us; it is a matter of us connecting with it.

In Aboriginal spirituality, when our life's journey aligns with our life purpose, we are on the path to contentment. Our spirituality tells us that to find this personal path we need to connect with a bigger path, the Dreaming Path.

The Dreaming Path has been there from the beginning for us to follow. It is about how each of us fulfills our responsibility to care for our place and all things in our place, including each other. How we do this will differ from person to person because we all have different stories, but if we are following the Dreaming Path, we are united and heading in the same direction. I don't see a lot of that right now.

Part of our personal story is therefore about contributing to a bigger story—that of community well-being. In addition to supporting increased individual well-being, this book aims to support the generation of stronger, vibrant communities that are incubators of well-being in mind, body, and spirit. As part of this vision, it is our hope that leaders—whether they be local, regional, national, or global—better understand and fulfill their responsibilities to care for their place and all things in their place above all other things. If they do, we all win.

The Dreaming Path is a book for all people. All that is required is an open mind and willingness to contemplate and reflect. It is about providing individuals and society with a different way of thinking that can inspire new perspectives on and commitments to achieving a better internal and external world.

More specifically, if you connect to any of the categories below, this book will be of value to you:

- an individual who wants to achieve increased purpose, meaning, and contentment in their life
- someone concerned about a friend or family member who you think is lost
- a person involved in a community service organization
- a person involved in developing government social policy
- a student interested in personal and community well-being
- someone who is passionate about preserving the natural environment
- an employee in the health and welfare sectors
- an educator
- a parent
- a leader
- someone passionate about reducing racism and inequality

In writing this book, Uncle Paul and I haven't attempted to give you prescriptive, guaranteed solutions to well-being. What we have tried to do is give you things to think about, just as if you were sitting around the fire yarning with us. How you use what we share is up to you.

Each chapter of this book reviews key themes that can help

you connect to the Dreaming Path, and in doing so, create and maintain improved well-being for yourself and the broader community. Key themes include the following:

- the importance of story
- relationships
- sharing
- unity
- love
- gratitude
- humility
- learning
- truth
- inspiration
- resilience
- being present
- healing from the past
- contentment
- responsibility
- leadership

The first two chapters provide an overview of Aboriginal spirituality, and the remainder of the book provides insights and thoughts that you can use in a practical way in your daily life. The book also prompts you, at times, to reflect on how you can use what you have learned to help others achieve improved well-being.

Each chapter of this book starts with a Dreamtime story. The word *dream* when describing traditional Aboriginal stories can be misleading, as it gives an impression of mythical, fairy-tale content that is disconnected from reality and therefore not that useful in day-to-day life. Dreamtime stories (often told through Aboriginal art, dance, and sites as well as orally) can appear to be very simple at first glance but in reality are multifaceted in terms of their messaging, multilayered in terms of their audience, and multipurpose in terms of their application. Each story can create meaningful conversation and learning, whether it is shared with a child, teenager, adult, or older person.

Dreamtime stories are Aboriginal parables designed to provide clear learning and guidance on key elements and rules that underpin the Lore. They are road maps for a life of increased purpose through improved understanding of personal values and responsibilities.

Throughout this book there are exercises for you to do should you choose to. They are there to help you better understand critical concepts and reflect on specific points of view. They aren't compulsory, so please don't feel guilty if you don't want to do a particular exercise—or any exercises, for that matter. Making your way through our words is meant to be fluid, not forced. This book aims to help you see life as less of a chore, so the last thing we want to do is create chores.

You will also find there are questions for you to consider. Like the exercises, they are optional: respond to them only if you choose to.

At the end of each chapter, important messages are provided. The messages capture the essence of each chapter's contents. They provide points of reference for you to reflect on long after you have finished reading this book. One or two of them might even become important notes to remind you of aspects of your life you would like to work on.

As you read this book, it is important to reflect on comments and concepts that resonate, but at the same time, try not to over-think any of it—that is not the Aboriginal way of learning. As you learn about our culture, you will hopefully start to realize that our way of life is about flowing with what is around us. So . . . as you read, flow with the words and thoughts, as you do when you are watching a movie. Enjoy the journey without worrying too much about the destination: trust that what you need will be given to you when you need it.

Many of the concepts we share will seem simple and common-sense. Don't let this fool you. What might seem to be a simple insight or comment could create a ripple of newfound awareness, understanding, and commitment that can change your life. That is what happened to me.

This time of reflection is about you, for you. Reflection and growth are two of the most important things you can do for your-self, so there's no need to rush. Take your time and don't be afraid to come back to different parts of the book to reread and do more reflection. You are worth it!

Uncle Paul and I hope you find these pages challenging, reward-ing, and affirming. We hope reading *The Dreaming Path* will ignite a thirst to listen to the perspectives of other Aboriginal people as well as the perspectives of other Indigenous and non-Indigenous peoples.

We are but two voices in the world choir. We need and wel-come other voices to join us. We look forward to you helping us create something new from something old . . . there is no time like the present to start!

In our stories, everything started from Country and our people went out throughout the world, and over time their skin changed, language changed, Lore was forgotten.

In 1788, some of the forgotten children came back.

Now, children, you are home. You need to awaken and listen to your Elders.

It is time for you to learn what you have lost.

—UNCLE PAUL GORDON

Chapter 1

Caring for Our Place
(The Importance of Story)

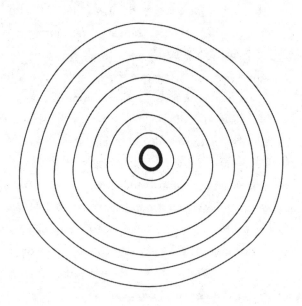

All things have spirit. We are all one.

The universe is a living being. We are all part of it. Everything has spirit and everything is connected.

When someone or something passes, where does it go? It goes back to where it came from and begins again. Nothing is ever lost: just missed until it is found again. We are one with all things. We all came from the same beginning.

When the world was conceived in the belly of the universe, the universe ate many things. The earth was being fed in readiness for birth.

Once, the earth was covered entirely by water, but under the water was our Mother, Gunni. The rainbow serpent, Wawaii, was inside Gunni's belly deep under the water. Then Wawaii started to move inside Gunni and she awoke and the land rose up out of the sea.

Wawaii brought the water from the ocean to the land, but as we know, salt water is not good for the land. So Wawaii took the salt out of the water and put the salt deep down in the soil and brought the fresh water to the top of the soil in things like springs. Wawaii traveled the country putting fresh water in special places throughout the land.

When Biamii, our sky father, looked down and saw our beautiful Mother rise from the ocean, he came down from the sky and they shared their love and made love and the first children were born. They were great ancestral animal beings that walked Country making mountains, valleys, and all the landscapes we can see today. It was a long process and there are many stories of how plants came to be, how animals came to be, how fish came to be, how birds came to be, how insects came to be, and so on. The creation of all things is linked back to our Mother, our Father, and Wawaii, the rainbow serpent.

Humans were the last ones to be made, and we came from the animal ancestors that were here before us. Every creature and every thing—whether it be animal, bird, insect, or plant—has story and Lore that connects us all. The sky, the sun, the moon, and the stars all have story and Lore as well. The Lore and the related stories explain the oneness and connectedness of all things. There is no separation between spirituality and everyday life. Everything is connected. Every action in our everyday life is connected back to the Lore.

The earth has all the emotions we have. Throughout her life, her emotions, illnesses, and loves have created the world we are now a part of. Our actions are not isolated. Everything we do impacts the earth and all things. Everything we do impacts what we are leaving for our children.

Academics generally believe that humans migrated to North America between 15,000 and 20,000 years ago while some archaeological evidence suggests this may have occurred more than 20,000 years ago. Scientific assessments of how long Aboriginal people have occupied the continent known as Australia vary from 50,000 to 120,000 years depending on what research is accessed.

From an Aboriginal cultural perspective, our Old People say we have been here since the beginning. Our creation stories reflect this belief and provide insight into how all living things, including Aboriginal people, came to exist in their traditional Country.

Our Old People also tell us that in the time before invasion, Aboriginal people lived rewarding and contented lives—physically, mentally, and spiritually.

Imagine a world where people have all they need to be contented. Where they live to be old and are happy in mind, body, and spirit. That is the way our people lived for a very, very long time. Life could sometimes be hard, but our knowledge of the land meant that we always had what we needed.

Throughout Australia, all aspects of traditional Aboriginal life have always been guided by the Lore. As explained earlier, this English word captures the concept of traditional knowledge that is passed on generationally.

In Australia, the words Dreamtime *and* Dreaming *are sometimes used to describe ancient stories that explain the Lore. There are even books that use the words* myths, legends, *and* fables *in their titles when referring to Dreamtime stories, and that is wrong. Our stories aren't myths or legends or fables—they aren't about dreams either. To us they are very real.*

In my language we use the word Ngurrampaa. Ngurrampaa is a better way of talking about the Dreamtime. Basically, it means "my relationship with my place and everything in my place." So the Lore is very much about what is my connection

with everything in my place and my Country. It is about how we
all connect with our place and everything in our place.

In the traditional Aboriginal world, everything—every
different species, type of rock, animal, reptile, and person—has
a story. A story of how it came to be. When you have a story
then you also have a song, and when you have a song you also
have a dance. They are all part of the one thing. By listening
to the different stories and understanding their lessons, we are
better able to care for our place and everything in our place
and connect to the Dreaming Path.

Story was critical in traditional Aboriginal people's lives as a vehicle of communication and as a means of sharing knowledge. From the day you were born, you were taught through story the importance of your surroundings and to connect with and respect those surroundings. Aboriginal people sometimes describe this as connecting with "their place" or "their Country." From an Aboriginal spiritual and cultural perspective, "your Country" or "your place" is pivotal to who you are. It is central to your existence. Country for an Aboriginal person is the place your ancestors were born, where they walked the land, where they went back to the land, and where they now walk the land as spirits. Country is where you connect in mind and spirit as you walk the earth, and where your body will be placed once you no longer walk this earth.

In our way, we belong to the land . . . it owns us; we don't own it. In our physical form, the land keeps us alive for the short time we are here . . . so we must respect it and ensure the footprints we leave do not harm it. The Mother is so beautiful to us that when our life in physical form is over, we may choose to return to our Country in spirit form so we can continue to care for Mother Earth and all of her children.

The Lore teaches us that all people who live on this land have a responsibility to love and care for it . . . regardless of where they were born. The first step in doing this is to connect with the land. Once you start doing this, you might be surprised how much better you feel about yourself and your life.

Exercise: Connecting with Place 1

Is there a place in the natural landscape where you just love being? The aim of this exercise is to help you connect with it.

It might help if you record the following words so you can listen to them with your eyes closed, or perhaps have someone read this script to you.

Let the chatter of your mind slip into the background. There are always things to think about in the now, but for the moment, you can let it all disappear.

As your mind begins to let go, start to picture a place you love. A place where you feel relaxed and in no rush to do anything. A place where you can just float in a bubble of peace . . . where there are no demands on you . . . where you can escape from everything for a little while. This place might be surrounded by stone, it might be sandy, it might be grassy. It might be in the mountains, it might be on the coast, it might be in the desert.

With all the time in the world, look around you. What can you see? You might notice lots of things in fine detail or you might just take in a blur of images.

Take your time and just absorb the living mural of nature. Right now, in this present moment, all these things are there for you to enjoy.

With all the time in the world, close your eyes and let your breath calmly flow in and out of your body, naturally and easily.

When you are ready, with your eyes still closed, notice what you can hear around you.

Take your time and enjoy the music of nature. Right now, in this present moment, all these things are there for you to enjoy. As you notice your breath once again, feel the peace and calm that is flowing through you. Stay with this feeling for a little while. Bathe in it as you would a hot, sudsy bath on a cold winter's afternoon.

When you are ready, look around you once again and notice how truly beautiful this place is.

Allow yourself to smile in wonder and gratitude if it feels right. Smile with your face. Smile with your eyes. Smile from a place deep inside.

Now reach out and connect with your surroundings.

Reach out with your heart.

Reach out with your mind.

Reach out with your spirit.

Connect with it all. There is no right or wrong way to do this ... just go with whatever feels right for you ... and as you do, feel the love and acceptance that surrounds you.

This place is for you. It will nurture you. It will care for you.

It will heal you.

Feel the calm yet profound power of this place. It will always give you all it has, unconditionally. Love, warmth, solace, strength, peace, protection, respite. All these things are there for you.

Now let your mind and spirit connect even more deeply with this place. Connect beyond what you can see or hear. Connect with the spirit of the tree. Connect with the spirit of the stone. Connect with the spirit of the water. As you do, feel the connection and love flow through your entire being.

Stay with this feeling for as long as you choose. There is no such thing as time: allow yourself the freedom to just be.

When you are ready . . . gently and in no particular rush . . . let the connection go and, in your own time, come back to the now.

How do you feel? How did you feel during the exercise? If you felt a sense of peace or perhaps joy or perhaps love, from an Aboriginal perspective you have connected with Country.

In Aboriginal spirituality, it is our responsibility to care for our place and all things in our place: this is both our collective and individual priority. This spiritual directive also has a practical significance.

If an individual was dependent on a machine every day of their life to survive, do you think they would take an interest in learning about how to use and maintain the machine so it didn't break down? Would they place a very high value on the machine?

The answer would more than likely be yes. The individual would do whatever was necessary to keep themselves safe.

The land gives life and maintains life for all of us and has done so since creation. We need to ensure it continues to do so. A cornerstone of Aboriginal life therefore has always been learning about the natural environment, passing on that knowledge and ensuring the land is cared for.

Traumatizing the land, including the sea and sky, contradicts the Lore. Harming the land is not following the obligation of caring for my place.

If you look back at the old ancient pagan beliefs of England, Ireland, Scotland, or France, you will find there was a time when people loved the land, looked after the land, and got their medicine and food from the land.

It was one big Lore once upon a time, right across the world. But somewhere in time something happened. Something happened in other parts of the world which stopped people from believing in the old ways.

They didn't respect the land the way they used to. But that doesn't mean the need to respect the land is not there today, because all of us human beings who live on this earth have only one earth to live on. If we don't learn to love it, and respect it and look after it the way we used to, then it will eventually die. Aboriginal spirituality is here for everybody and anybody who wants to be able to connect to their place and to their Mother, the land.

If people want to come and connect to Country, Aboriginal people like myself are always willing to share and teach how to. We can help people from all parts of the world bring back their old ways and connect with their Old Ones. The earth gives us life. We need to make sure we look after it.

It is important to understand that the Lore belongs to the land, not the people. The fabric of caring for place is woven into the desert sands. It is in the mountains, in the waters, in the forests, in the ground, and in the sky.

> *People often tell me how sad it is our culture is gone. Our culture isn't gone at all. We are still here . . . and the stories themselves are part of the land . . . are in the land. They will be still in the land long after I am gone. Every person who lives on this land has a responsibility to listen to it, understand it, and care for it in accordance with the Lore.*

In traditional times, no action or activity was above the Lore. Anyone breaking the Lore would be causing potential harm and suffering to the land and/or things that belonged to the land. Breaking the Lore therefore had serious consequences.

When we watch the world news, or as we read our social media feeds from around the world, do you think human beings as a global entity are following the essence of the Lore? That is, do you think human beings as a collective are "caring for their place and all things in their place" above all other things?

How does the modern world view the land? Is it in the background of the theater of life or is it the main stage? Do we live to serve it or do we expect it to serve us? In order to answer this question, consider the change in the earth's population over the past two hundred years. In that time, the population has grown from 1 billion to more than 7.7 billion. Some people would argue that this increase is a fairly natural result of exponential growth, and they may be right. But from an Aboriginal perspective, the number of people now living on this earth is an indication of the Lore being broken and people as a collective placing themselves above the earth and nature. Our Old People might say, "If there are too many people living in one place, they will eventually destroy the balance of that place. You silly people are now acting as if the earth is here to serve you when it should be the other way around. You are here to serve it."

Of the more than 7.7 billion people who are on this earth, how many are committed to spending every minute of their lives caring for the land? Is the land something we feel owns us (as is the case with Aboriginal people) or is it an asset/resource to be bought, sold, drilled, cut, mined, poisoned, cleared, controlled, and conquered?

I have a degree in business, have lectured in economics, and have run a corporation with a $70 million Australian annual budget, so I understand capitalist market forces and the importance of employment, agriculture, industry, and trade in supporting our current world population. We cannot go back to a population of a billion people, and in many ways, traditional land management practices are no longer workable in a world with land titles, fences, cities, and the need for continuous economic growth. At the same time, there is still much to be learned by bringing the two worlds together. We certainly cannot continue our destructive ways.

In traditional times, Aboriginal kinship and governance systems controlled the number of people living on Country to ensure the land could provide for the population in a sustainable way. For instance, in the Country of my people, the Worimi people, men would ingest a natural contraceptive made from a plant extract when hard times, such as a drought, were imminent, to ensure the population didn't grow beyond what the land could sustain.

Controlling population growth is obviously contentious, but an important learning from the Aboriginal worldview is the over-arching need to care for the planet. This means supporting the current population with employment, agricultural, industry, and trade practices that nurture the environment rather than destroy it. There is no doubt the world has the collective genius to do this; what seems to be currently missing is the aggregate will.

In traditional times, children were taught to love the land and all things connected to the land.

> As a child, we are given many, many Ngurrampaa stories. From the stories come morals and from the morals come the rules of the land and the rules of society. From the rules comes L-A-W law.

As soon as a child was born, they were immersed in the learning process through connection to story, including oral story, dance, song, and art. As the child grew, the stories were repeated again and again. As the child transitioned to puberty, they would know hundreds of stories that provided them with much of the knowledge and values they needed for an adult life of meaning and well-being.

The rite of initiation was the culmination of this part of the learning process and the milestone whereby a child became an adult and was given full adult responsibilities. Upon receiving these responsibilities, the individual was subject to the Lore, including punishment if the rules of the Lore were broken.

In our contemporary society, the requirement to follow the rules and consequent penalties for not adhering to them can be described as L-A-W law. These rules are usually developed in one of two ways: either through statute law (the law made by the legislature) or case law (based on the decision of judges in the superior courts). Contemporary laws are often hard to interpret and require specialized expertise in the form of lawyers.

Unlike traditional Aboriginal society, in which each young person knew every rule they had to live by, it is impractical to expect the contemporary school system to provide students with knowledge of the many rules they are expected to uphold. There is therefore no connection between L-O-R-E (knowledge) and L-A-W (rules).

In Aboriginal society, the connectivity of L-A-W (rules) to L-O-R-E (knowledge) has always been critical. L-O-R-E is a reflection of tens of thousands of years of traditional stories, the knowledge they provide, and the morals and responsibilities that are embedded in that knowledge.

Given the breadth of L-O-R-E as a learning system and its importance in establishing L-A-W in traditional Aboriginal society, it is no surprise that Aboriginal societal life was one of connectivity, harmony, and balance.

When you grew up in traditional Aboriginal society, you learned all about rocks. And sometimes Old People will say, "You know those rocks. They grow. Rocks are born, rocks get pregnant, rocks breathe, and rocks die like all things do."

So there are things other people might think are inanimate that Aboriginal people talk about as having spirit. Everything has spirit and soul and everything has the right to be respected. And everything has a story.

When you grow up learning all about these things, the more you know—the more stories you know—the more you understand your place. The stories tell you about bush tucker, bush medicine, the rules of your society, values, and magic.

So from a really, really early age, Aboriginal kids would sit down with all their relatives—their mothers, fathers, grandparents, aunties, uncles—and be told stories. And from these stories they were learning all their values.

And the more you learn about your place, the easier it is to exist in your place and the more you love your place. If you know where bush medicine is, or bush tucker is, or where shelter is, the easier it is to live in your place and connect with it. That place is where you come from. It is your place.

Your place gives you everything you need. It gives you water and it gives you food. It gives you shelter, it gives you medicine, and it gives you connection to one another.

And when you listen to the Old People, they will tell you, "Don't just listen to humans, listen to them old animal ancestors too. Listen to the kangaroos, listen to the emus, listen to the birds, listen to the witchetty grubs."

All things will teach you if you take notice. And the more things you take notice of, learn from, and have a connection to the more you understand and love what is around you.

So in Aboriginal society, all things were respected as equal. There was no "lesser" creature on earth. Everything had a right to exist and everything was connected to everything else.

In the Aboriginal worldview we are all equal. Plants, rocks, animals, insects, and everything around us is considered our teacher.

The more I connect to what is around me, the more I look at what is around me, the more I listen to what is around me, the more I will learn.

This connectivity is inherent in the Aboriginal L-O-R-E system, which is underpinned by unity, equality, and love. Non-Aboriginal law, by contrast, is a system underpinned by division, inequality, and fear that disconnects us from our surroundings. It is unlikely this book will overhaul the legal system, but it can hopefully motivate you to be part of a revitalization of the L-O-R-E system by increasing connectedness and learning through the sharing of story.

As adults, it is important for us to learn, create, and share as many stories as possible with our children and with each other and, thanks to modern technology, there is no reason we can't share those stories right across the world. We have all witnessed how quickly negative stories can flood the planet and how these stories drain us. The antidote is to do the same with positive stories (Ngurrampaa stories, real-life stories, creative stories) so we can feel inspired by the magnificence that is around us. There really is nothing stopping us.

Sharing positive stories and collectively celebrating the many great things happening all around us will mean we focus on what we have got rather than what we haven't. It will help us focus on what we have in common rather than our differences. By doing this, we can help create a more united, positive, and connected world of understanding, tolerance, and respect. By sharing stories, we are generating positive energy and magic in the world—and everyone benefits from that! The more positivity we generate, the more positivity we will receive—and the more magic we will begin to feel in our life.

It is important to note that celebrating the magic in the world is no excuse to shy away from the reality that there are bad things and injustices happening around us as well. By creating unity and trust, we are in a far better position to call out wrongs, engage in truth-telling, expose tokenism, and create authentic change in areas where change is very much needed.

For some people, life can be a challenge. Managing many competing priorities can wear us down. The cynic within us can dominate, making it hard to believe in magic and the power of story. The world can seem far too complex and hostile for the seemingly simplistic messages within the Lore to be relevant.

The Lore is very much relevant to people today. The old principles of caring for one another, looking after the place we live in, and being connected to the environment around us are just as relevant to us today as in traditional times. This is because without each other and without a healthy natural environment, what have we got?

And we need to tell our kids stories.

People today tell kids stories like "The Three Little Pigs" or "Cinderella." People think these are just fairy tales but they reveal useful morals to live by. What we need to think about is what do these stories mean? What values can they teach us? We need to teach our kids more and more the importance of story so they will understand things better.

By creating a world where we share and accept each other's stories without judgment or prejudice, by creating a world where each of us takes responsibility for our place and all things in our place, by creating a world where we share all that we have, we will see individuals, communities, regions, states, countries, continents, and the entire earth better able to achieve fulfillment and well-being.

Remember Neil Armstrong's famous words, "One small step for a man, one giant leap for mankind"? By each of us making the effort to care for our place and all things in our place, we might only be taking one small step individually, but we are doing something much greater collectively. If enough of us decide to take that one small step, humanity can take one giant leap.

The Lore is not for everybody, and some who don't have it find it hard to accept. But it is here for anyone who wants it.

The beauty and the power of the Lore is something we can all be part of. In creating this brave new world of common purpose, connectedness, and sharing, the importance of accepting others' stories, even if they contradict our own beliefs, cannot be emphasized enough.

I don't expect you to believe in what I believe in. But I expect you to respect what I believe in as I will respect what you believe in. To us, our Dreamtime stories are not fairy tales. To us these stories are real. They are traditional Lore stories and we believe in them. If I was to call the Bible a Dreamtime book, how would Christians feel? If I was to call the Koran a Dreamtime book, how would Muslims feel? Our stories are just as true and real to us as anybody else's story is to them.

How often do you tell stories? Do you share stories with kids? Do you share stories with adults? How often do you listen to stories? If you aren't including stories in your life, you are missing out on an opportunity to learn and grow.

Many years ago, I was employed in an executive role with TAFE (Technical and Further Education) New South Wales that involved, among other things, attendance at regular executive meetings. Following one of these meetings, a colleague told me that another colleague had said, "Here goes Paul. Telling another story again." I took this as a compliment.

My tendency to share information through story didn't seem to erode my career progression (not that I had career aspirations). Within a very short period I was promoted to CEO of a TAFE institute where I had responsibility for more than 1,200 staff and 23,000 students over ten campuses. In my third year in the role, our institute was awarded "Large Training Provider of the Year New South Wales" and short-listed to the top three for the Australian award. My experience was that storytelling can be a powerful vehicle of connection in a diverse range of settings. By sharing story, we are able to better connect to colleagues, family, friends, and strangers. By listening to traditional Aboriginal story, we are able to better connect to spirit and to the land.

In Aboriginal culture, the land—the Mother—is the most beautiful thing in the universe. Our Mother gives us everything we need to live a good life, just like a human mother provides everything the unborn child needs to live and grow in the womb.

If I learn all I can about my Mother . . . if I sing for her . . . if I dance for her . . . if I love her . . . if I care for her . . . she will always give me what I need.

When British occupation commenced in Australia in 1788, the boat people had no understanding or desire to understand Aboriginal people's connection to the land and the many systems they had in place to sustain the land. The lack of houses and farms (or at least anything the British recognized as houses and farms) fueled the misconception of *terra nullius* (land belonging to no one). Many of the new arrivals saw Aboriginal people as nothing more than wild animals and held a view that the sooner Aboriginal people died out, the better.

Had the new arrivals built relationships instead of armies—listened to the people born of this land and learned from them—the past two hundred and thirty years of Australian history, and current-day Australia, would be a far different story. Instead of a story of invasion, massacres, murder, disease, dislocation, pain, loss, trauma, and disadvantage for Aboriginal people, there would be a story of collaboration, life, respect, growth, celebration, and equality. It isn't too late to reshape the next chapters of this story.

The creation of new relationships between Aboriginal and non-Aboriginal people can't change the past but it can address the past. This is an exciting time. A new platform can be created across the world: a platform of mutual understanding and respect that can allow the global story to become a unified one. With understanding, love, and purpose, we can create a better world story.

At the moment, the global story incorporates a number of good-news items, such as technological advancement, medical breakthroughs, and social initiatives that are positively impacting the lives of many people in parts of the world. At the same time, there are still significant incidences of poverty, hunger, homelessness, sickness, incarceration, crime, and lack of access to basic services for specific groups of people. While this "social failure" exists, we are not supporting good individual stories and not creating a good global story.

To enable the world to create the best story possible, we need honest reflection and a genuine desire to overcome disadvantage in all its forms. If every nation was to commit to caring for its place and all things in their place, social failure would no longer exist. Environmental failure would also be reduced.

Some people might argue that there have always been winners and losers in life and that disadvantage is an unfortunate reality in society, but that kind of thinking is not caring or compassionate and doesn't reflect our true capacity to achieve greatness if we are brave enough to demand it. Creating a better story for ourselves and the planet is not a fantasy. Numerous experts suggest there are plenty of resources—food, water, housing—more than enough for everyone. The resources are there, if we are willing to reshape our approach to distributing them. Change is a very real possibility if we want to make it happen. To create a better world for all people, we need change.

If, like me, you believe human-induced climate change is real then you will agree that we need to find new ways of living. If we are willing to look, listen, and be honest with ourselves, we know that things are not right. As a collective, we are failing in our responsibilities to each other and the earth.

Everything that keeps us alive comes from the earth. The Mother continues to give us all we need, even though we don't collectively sing for her, dance for her, love her, or care for her as we once did.

Aboriginal spiritual belief and spiritual Lore is a law of responsibility to all things. When we look at Western law, we see it is based on a platform of rights. People believe they have the right to do what they like, providing it sits within the Western law system. I see people time and time again going out and doing things because they have the right to, without any thought about their responsibilities. Action that is based on rights with no connection to responsibility undermines the Lore. When Lore is broken, there will always be consequences. If we believe the land is a gift from God, then why don't we look after it so it is still the way God presented it to us? When we buy a child a toy and the child breaks it, we say that the child has done the wrong thing. The land is far more precious than a child's toy and we should all feel a responsibility to care for it.

With a rights mindset, people say they have the right to cut down trees, they have the right to dig the land up, they have the right to treat the earth as a commodity—to buy and sell, to do with it as they want. But who gave them that right? And where does responsibility lie?

I have had the privilege of accessing formal education and cultural education in my life. Both systems have given me critical insights and skills I use on a daily basis.

My degree in business, diplomas in surveying and drafting, PhD in Creative Practice, and postgraduate studies in leadership, executive coaching, and governance have given me many skills that I am grateful for but my greatest learning has been through my twenty-plus years spent with cultural Elders. The knowledge they have given me has provided me with an unshakable belief in the applicability, importance, and transferability of traditional Aboriginal cultural knowledge to the modern world. Bringing the two worlds together will benefit us all and, more important, enable the planet to disinfect and heal so future generations can immerse themselves in the diversity and abundance that Mother Earth has to share with us.

By enacting urgent actions to better care for our place, we can prevent further damage to the planet and ourselves. We have a greater capacity to do this than some might think.

Far too often, across the world we hear about natural and human-generated catastrophes that give rise to indescribable hardship, pain, suffering, and grief. It is in these times of darkness we often see the light of humanity and spirit shine the brightest. We see footage showing stories of courage and kindness and hear accounts of miracles that inspire us to believe that things can get better . . . that give us hope. No matter how dark an event can be, in time, with patience and predictability, nature will begin to reshape the landscape, healing and renewing Country, reminding us the cycle of life and is never ending. From the ashes of despair, a phoenix of renewal can rise if we unite with each other and nature. During these times of catastrophe, we have demonstrated that as a collective we can quickly adapt when the need is compelling. We can use this superpower to change the world for the better, if our desire is strong enough.

No matter what kind of hardship you might be facing in life, you are also able to reflect and renew. You have the power within to make whatever changes are necessary to no longer feel like you are going around in circles. By connecting to nature and caring for what is around you, you are on your way to finding the

Dreaming Path. The following chapters will show you how to follow it in a way that recognizes, respects, and harnesses your unique qualities so that you can walk your footsteps with independence, purpose, confidence, and belief.

Message 1

Care for your place and all things in your place.

Message 2

Everything and everyone has a story. The more stories we share, the more we learn. The more we learn, the more we grow.
The more we grow, the closer we are to achieving well-being—individually and universally.

Chapter 2

Relationships, Sharing, and Unity

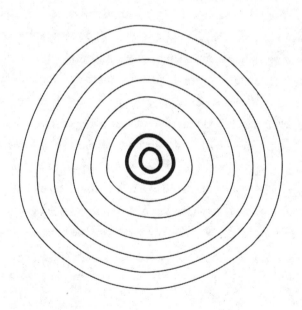

A little while after the diniwan (emu chicks) had hatched, their father took them for a walk to show them what to gather and eat. He also showed them the things they shouldn't eat.

Their Country was still untouched by the white-skinned people who appeared with the white sails on the water, so the bush was alive with the movement and sound of all kinds of life.

Throughout the day, the emu chicks met many of their clan. They met members of their bundar (kangaroo) family, thikarbilla (echidna) family, and their googar (goanna) family.

As the father emu walked toward different animals with the chicks following close behind, they heard many animals say, "Wow, here comes our family." It made the chicks feel very special. It also made them wonder.

Toward the end of what had been a very exciting day, one of the chicks asked their father, "Why are all these animals our family? They don't look like us but they feel like us."

"Sit down and listen, children," the father replied. They found a big shady tree by a creek and sat down. The chicks looked up at their father, their small fluffy wings shaking with excitement.

"A long time ago, in the beginning of the Ngurrampaa, there were two rainbow snakes."

The chicks started to get even more excited. They loved hearing stories, but they especially loved hearing stories about the rainbow snakes.

"The rainbow snakes were very clever—way smarter than us. They often laughed at us because of the way we lived. Our lives weren't like they are now, when we care for our place and all things in our place. Back then, we didn't really get on very well because we didn't understand the importance of relationships.

"One day a little boy said to the rainbow snakes, 'Why do you laugh at us and judge us? If you have knowledge that we do not have, why don't you share that with us. Please teach us.'

"The snakes were impressed with the little boy. 'Yes. That is a good idea. We will share with you. Do you know you are all the same?' they said. 'You have all come from the same place, from the land—our Mother. You are all family. If you all sit down and talk to each other . . . If you all sit down and share stories . . . you will realize that your stories are all a little bit different but they are also the same.

"'All the stories say we should love one another; we should share and not steal from one another; we should tell the truth and not lie to each other. So sit down and share stories. Once you do this, you will learn about how important family is and how to care for each other. You will learn the importance of relationships.'"

The emu chicks nodded as their father spoke. "We understand now," they said in one voice.

"But there is more to share," the father emu said. "Over the many thousands of years since the snakes shared with us the importance of relationships, we have shared story, attended each other's ceremonies, married one another, and cared for one another. We have no armies, no forts, no castles, no fences like the new people who have come to this

place. We don't need these things because we are all one with
each other and we are all one with the land. We are all family.
You all have grandmothers, grandfathers, mothers, fathers,
brothers, and sisters. You will meet them all as you grow."

The bush had become quiet. Other animals had come to
listen to the father speak. The father was happy with the
chance to share story with the mob.

"And one day, when you are older, you will marry someone
who is not part of your family and, from that relationship,
over time, they will also become family. But that is another
story. Everyone is family, so as you grow, love them, share
with them, and never hurt them, and they will do the same."

That night, as the emu chicks were about to go to sleep,
they shared the story of their day. They all agreed how lucky
they were to have so many relations and how they looked
forward to meeting more and more of their family. But that,
too, is another story. In fact, it is many stories.

Psychology literature suggests that human beings are herd
animals. We survive only in highly coordinated groups. Individually, we are designed to pick up social cues and coordinate
and align our behavior with that of those around us so we can
fit in. Recent research supports this premise, finding that fitting
in with those around us soothes us while social disapproval pro-
vokes the brain's danger circuits and can create agitation. Relationships are therefore an inherent component of well-being.

The creation and maintenance of relationships has been a cornerstone of Aboriginal culture since the beginning—with stories,

dance, song, and art reinforcing the importance of connection between all things.

The creation story at the beginning of Chapter 1 tells us how all things were conceived from the Mother and Father's love and born of the one Mother. All living things—the birds, trees, plants, fish, insects, animals, humans, and so on—are family.

The creation story also tells us that human beings were the last to be created. We are the youngest siblings in the family of living things. As the youngest, we are told to remember that everything around us is older and wiser than us. Our brothers and sisters are our teachers and we should never place ourselves above them. The Old People say that if we want to gain true wisdom, our greatest learning happens when we take ourselves into the bush and spend time with our family. They say that if we are able sit quietly, look at and listen to what is around us (that is, no phone, books or other people to distract us), we will be given more knowledge (conscious and unconscious) than we thought possible.

Aboriginal culture acknowledges the importance of human relationships, but also tells us that our responsibilities are far broader than to each other. We must also build relationships with our place and all things in our place.

Exercise: Connecting with Place 2

Get a blank piece of paper and something to write with.

Draw a rough map of where you live, with your residence at the center. Don't worry about perfection. Whatever you draw will be perfect for this exercise.

Draw an approximate circle on the map that represents the geographic area you feel connected to. The circle might have a radius of one mile, ten miles, or one hundred miles. It doesn't matter how big the circle is. What really matters is that the circle reflects the natural landscape you feel part of.

Close your eyes and scan the landscape in your circle. As you do, one by one, notice the natural features that inspire you. There might be streams, rivers, parks, mountains, forests, grass plains, desert plains, or other places that are special to you. As you zoom in on each natural feature, connect with it and let this place welcome you. Feel the joy of this place flow through you as you allow yourself to become part of it.

Stay with each place as long as you choose. There is no such thing as time as you allow your spirit to soar for a little while.

When you have visited enough places in your circle of connection and when you are ready . . . gently and in no particular rush . . . let the connection to the last image go and in your own time come back to the now.

How do you feel? How did you feel during the exercise?

Reflect on the places you visited and identify three places in your circle that you will physically visit on a regular basis. Once you have identified them, create a "visitation plan," including dates, and commit to it.

Connecting with Country, whether it be in your mind or physically, in some ways reflects the popular modern practice of mindfulness, which involves being present and fully engaged with experiences occurring in the present moment. It is also much more than that. Connecting with Country and those things that live in Country allows us to reconnect with our broader family and feel their love and nurture.

Connecting with Country enables us to:

- have time for ourselves;
- embrace quiet for a little while;
- allow ourselves to just be;
- let go of anxiety;
- reenergize and renew;
- remember how special we are;
- be thankful; and
- share love, respect, and humility with what is around us.

Think about a time when you might have been feeling stressed or overwhelmed and when you intuitively or perhaps consciously sought solace in nature. The feeling of release you triggered by going back to nature was much more than a physical reaction to the peace and quiet you felt you needed.

In our way of believing, by allowing the organic flow of nature to surround you and by letting go of the omnipresent, mechanistic rush of the Western world, you are allowing yourself to connect with the "inner you," the "wise you," the "authentic you" that can be so easily drowned out by the noise of the "getting-things-done you."

You are allowing yourself to connect with something much bigger than you . . . much older than you . . . much wiser than you. You are connecting with spirit and with your family, your relatives that Mother Earth gave birth to so long ago. By connecting with your spiritual family, you are engaged in a symbiotic healing process, a mutually beneficial relationship that has little cost and major benefits.

If you close your eyes and just let the thought of sharing mutual healing with a special place in Country wash through you, you might feel how right this suggestion feels. If you do, congratulations on connecting with your "intuitive self." Building on this connection will provide you with insight and learning that might surprise you. Trusting the advice your intuitive self provides will change your life in a powerful and positive way. Building this relationship with yourself is the first step on the path of improved well-being.

In our way, our "intuitive self" is also our "ancient self."

When a baby is born, that soul has been here for a long time, maybe forever. It could have chosen to come back as a spirit or as something else, but it has chosen to come back as a physical body again. The parents and that community now have the responsibility of ensuring they give this baby the support, guidance, and learning it needs to achieve its life purpose, its Dreaming.

When a person dies, as we all must, death is the beginning of another long journey back to the spirit world, and, while that spirit is on that journey, the people left behind do not say the name of that person until they have completed their journey. It could be up to one or two years until that name can be spoken again.

Once the journey of the spirit is completed, their name can be spoken again, which will allow their spirit to come back into the physical world if it chooses to. It is a cycle of renewal like all things have a cycle of renewal.

After we pass away in physical form, the spirit returns to the Spirit Pool and our body goes back to the Mother, where our flesh and fluid returns to the physical environment. Our body becomes part of the earth's nutrient supply while our water (which is around 60 percent of our body) leaves our body and becomes part of the water cycle.

Over time, the water that was once part of our body, through transpiration, runoff, filtration, and precipitation, is absorbed by plants and consumed by animals. We become part of them. As the cycle repeats over time, we become part of all things. We are timeless.

When we connect with the environment through activities such as the Connecting with Place exercises, not only are we connecting with family, we are also connecting with our infinite self.

Aboriginal culture, stories, and knowledge also incorporate the sky and stars. There are stories of the emu; stories of the turkey; stories of the bad clever man; stories of the dancing man; stories of the loving grandmother; stories of the child who fell to earth; and stories of the seven sisters. There are stories that tell us about meteors that have fallen and stardust that has descended on earth since the beginning—becoming part of the natural environment as we are. Over time, we have become part of the universe.

In the Aboriginal way, when we look around Country during the day, we are surrounded by things we have a relationship with. When we look to the sky at night, it is the same. Even in our darkest times, when we might feel alone and unloved, we are surrounded by relationships—we are surrounded by a universe of love. These connections are essential components of our well-being, as is our connection to other people.

As we engage in day-to-day life, we manage a number of personal relationships in a range of contexts, including family, community, work, sport, and social settings. The effectiveness of these relationships depends on a number of factors:

- commitment
- communication
- trust
- honesty
- respect
- intimacy
- shared values
- realistic expectations
- understanding
- equality
- empathy

Maintaining a good relationship therefore requires commitment and effort. It starts with understanding the other person's story and related needs.

Our stories and our needs are extremely diverse, of course, but they have a degree of commonality at different stages in our lives. A review of the traditional Aboriginal life cycle provides us with some cultural perspectives on the aging process and our needs as we move from baby to child to adolescent to young adult to parent to grandparent to elderly person.

BIRTH: As we grow in the womb and immediately after birth, our story is all before us. The servicing of our needs often relies on our physical mother providing food for us and our family providing us with shelter and nurture. Our relationships dictate whether we live or die.

In traditional Aboriginal society, birth was a significant event that generated a sacred ceremony and large-scale celebrations.

From the day a baby was born, kinship relationships would be established. If it was a boy, he might be recognized as a grandfather, or a father, or a big brother, a baby brother, or an uncle. If the baby was a girl, she might be recognized as a grandmother, or a mother, a big sister, a baby sister, or an aunt under what we called our "skin system." From day one, everybody old enough to understand would know their obligations and responsibilities to that child because of the connection through their skin system.

In addition to being biologically sacred, the relationship between mother and child was also considered spiritually sacred, given we are all children of Mother Earth. Both the human mother and the land—the Mother—conceive, give birth to, and nurture life. Without the Mother and without mothers, life cannot exist. There are numerous Aboriginal engravings, tens of thousands of years old, that contain stories teaching us these two things and highlighting the importance of respecting women.

Think about the world as a whole. Do you think there is global consistency in terms of respect and responsibility for motherhood and care for the newborn child?

The reality is that the spiritual, universal sacredness of new life does not necessarily translate into an equal chance of survival in different parts of the world: 2.5 million children died in the first month of life in 2018, many from poverty-related issues. The world is in a state of imbalance if the likelihood of a child living to five years of age is related to the particular socioeconomic conditions into which they might be born. This state of affairs didn't exist in traditional Aboriginal society, given there was no such thing as socioeconomic disadvantage and therefore no such thing as poverty-related infant mortality.

Is the birth of a child celebrated by the community you live in? What do you think are your responsibilities to a child born into your family or extended family? What do you think are your responsibilities to a child born in your street or suburb? What do you think are your responsibilities to a child born on the other side of the world?

CHILD: As a baby transitions to toddler and beyond, their needs broaden from safety, security, and stability to include emotional connection, relationships love, and structure. The learning process creates the space into which the child will grow, and so is critical in this stage of their life. If we are given the right learning, our older years can flow easily. If we are given the wrong learning, our older years can become extremely difficult. In traditional times, the learning process was an integrated amalgam of story, play, and experiential activities. Childhood was a time of curiosity, joy, connection, and love as the child formed relationships with everything that surrounded them.

Many of the stories told to children involved imaginative and larger-than-life imagery intended to entertain so that memory retention was maximized. Storytelling took place outdoors, surrounded by significant places and objects that enriched the process.

There was a little lizard who couldn't stop eating. He wanted to eat everything. He started off eating small things, then as he grew he started to eat bigger things. He started off very small, about as long as a pinky finger. But he ate and he ate and he ate and he ate until, one day, he was as big as a whale. And still he kept eating. One day, he ate a snake, two fish, a woman, and a big kangaroo. When the kangaroo was inside the lizard's belly and saw the snake, fish, and woman still alive, the kangaroo started to jump up and down and said, "I will kick and I will kick on the side of the lizard's belly and get us out of here."

The lizard felt the pains in his stomach, just like we do when we eat too much, and started to worry. The kangaroo jumped and jumped and jumped until the lizard's belly burst and the kangaroo, the woman, the snake, and two fish were free.

That lizard was then punished and turned into a big rock.

This rock is next to a creek and you can walk up to it and see it looks like a lizard. At the side of the big rock facing the creek there is a cave. When you look into the cave you can see drawings of the fish, snake, and woman. Those drawings have been there for thousands of years. Across from the cave there is also a smaller rock with marks on it that look like kangaroo footprints. This smaller rock is the part of the lizard's belly that was kicked out by the kangaroo and landed on the other side of the creek.

This story is told to stop children from eating too much and from eating the wrong things, because if you do, you will have a very sick belly like the lizard. Now the lizard is in the landscape as a rock. It tells us why we should do the right thing. We should only ever eat what we need and not any more than that.

The Australian landscape is full of stories that we learn from.

Many stories for children focused on positive themes such as sharing, being respectful, being humble, and being loving. Although teaching responsibilities were shared throughout the community, grandparents were particularly important in this process.

Fear was also used to create learner engagement, maximize memory retention, and encourage the generation of desired behaviors. When sitting around the fire at night, the Old People would sometimes describe and act out colorful and terrifying accounts of mystical beings.

Since the beginning, kids have been told about the yurri. They were told the yurri is a little creature about one meter tall who is covered in hair, walks on two legs, is very strong, has big canine teeth, and sits out in the darkness away from the fire waiting for kids who wander away from camp.

They were told many stories of kids being taken away by a yurri (sometimes called the little hairy man). Quite often when the kids were playing in the firelight, the Old People would count the children and tell the children they were making sure there weren't extra kids playing in the game because the yurri would sometimes join in the play so they could take the kids away.

The kids knew they needed to stay within the firelight so the Old People could always see them. That way, no one had to worry about children becoming lost or hurt in the darkness. As children went through ceremony and became adults, more of the story of the yurri would be revealed.

The above story was told to ensure the safety of the child. As the child passed through initiation, the layers added to the story would shift the narrative from one of fear to one of deeper spiritual meaning. The fear of the dark would transition into an understanding of the dark, and the yurri would shift from figures of terror to figures of healing.

For more than 60,000 years, the rearing of a child was a community responsibility involving every single member. Being allowed to make mistakes was part of the learning process. A child's life was continually stimulating, full of play, full of learning, surrounded by story, and involved the continuing establishment and reinforcement of relationships. The learning process was focused on enabling each child to develop a strong sense of self in addition to preparing the child for an adult life where they had all they needed to fulfill their responsibilities and achieve well-being in mind, body, and spirit.

In our contemporary society, are our children supported, nurtured, and loved in a way where they are able to build a strong sense of self and have the learning they need to transition smoothly into an adult world of responsibility and well-being? Does their journey include the establishment of a broad range of relationships, which enables them to benefit from a diversity of experiences, knowledge bases, and support?

Given the narrow scope of many school curriculums, the amount of time many children spend engaged in technology and video games, the need in many instances for both parents to work, the decrease in extended family connectivity, and the difficulties in developing community networks, how do we ensure children are able to grow up in an environment that best prepares them for the journey ahead?

Think about your childhood. Did you have nurture, support, guidance, love, and care? If you did, how did it feel and how has it impacted your story so far? If you didn't, how did it feel and what impact did that have on your life?

I feel lucky when I look back on my early life, as my childhood years are filled with many fond memories. They are mainly around playing with my cousins on the Karuah Aboriginal Reserve (affectionately called "the Mish"). They were carefree days of play and laughter, where time didn't exist and the future was a concept that was alien to me.

TEENAGER/YOUNG ADULT: My transition from child to teenager to young adult was not as pleasant. The scars of being treated differently because I was Aboriginal, the scars of trying to fit in, the scars of being called a "boong" and a "dumb coon," the scars of well-intentioned people's expectations, the scars of wanting to be liked, and the trauma of multiple rejections (particularly from girls) became seeds of doubt that germinated and flourished in my later years, leading to acute anxiety and depression in my mid-thirties.

It is my belief that today's teenagers and young adults (Aboriginal and non-Aboriginal) face even more complex challenges and are more at risk of trauma than was the case in my time. The list below captures some, but not all, the issues young people can face each day:

- self-esteem
- body image
- stress and anxiety
- bullying
- depression
- cyber addiction
- drinking
- smoking
- drugs
- peer pressure
- competition
- academic pressure
- social media
- heartbreak
- poor sleep
- exposure to violence (television, film, and games)
- the casualized labor market
- high unemployment
- judgment from older generations

A plant will grow to its potential only if it is placed in the right soil and given the right nurturing. The above list highlights how many potential toxins there are that can infiltrate a young person's soil and the need for young people to have a substantial support network to help them get their soil right. If the soil is too barren or poisoned, their growth will be impaired and their adult life potentially more difficult.

In traditional times, many of the issues highlighted in the list did not exist. Preparing a young person for adult life in a way that embraced responsibility and fostered well-being in mind, body, and spirit was much easier than it is now.

This doesn't mean we can't learn from the past, including the importance of providing the right knowledge and support.

From puberty onward, young adults attended many ceremonies and continued to learn about their responsibilities and obligations to one another, their land, the creatures in their land, and the spiritual connections to all things.

Once the gift of knowledge was given, the responsibility of upholding that knowledge would be expected and reinforced. The little stories the young adults learned as a child stood them in good stead for their adult life.

Rite of passage to being an adult had to be earned—not expected just because of your age. For example, I have the right to go into a pub when I am eighteen. I can legally consent to sex when I am sixteen. I have the right to apply for a driver's license when I am seventeen. People can demand their rights but have they earned a particular right?

Aboriginal Lore is based on responsibility. You had no rights until you accepted the gift of responsibility. Is the eighteen-year-old responsible with their consumption of alcohol? Is the sixteen-year-old responsible with their sexual practices? Is the seventeen-year-old responsible with the way they drive their car?

In carrying out their responsibilities, young adults were never on their own. The entire community, including the Elders, were always there for them.

Although autonomy and the ability to walk your own footsteps is important in Aboriginal culture (by the age of twelve you had all the skills you needed to survive alone on the land), independence did not mean isolation or alienation.

In traditional times, as the individual became a young adult, preexisting relationships were maintained and in some ways escalated, given the young adult now had a formal responsibility to care for everyone in their community. Given there was no such thing as a forty-hour working week (or a mortgage), the individual had more than enough time to:

- carry out daily living activities (hunting, cooking, and survival-related activities took no more than one or two hours a day);
- maintain relationships;
- care for Country;
- care for all things on Country;
- care for community;
- participate in ceremony;
- engage in the learning process;
- fulfill other responsibilities; and
- practice good self-care.

The principle of lifelong learning was an intrinsic element of traditional culture and ensured that the young adult continued to build their knowledge base throughout their life. Traditional learning involved a hierarchy of skills similar in a way to current-day education frameworks (primary school, high school, college, university), although the learning purpose, learning content, teaching style, and educational context were completely different.

An important part of the traditional learning process was the totemic system. Totems themselves are a kinship connection between a person and an animal or plant in a way that is spiritually symbolic. Each individual had several totems and a responsibility to learn all there was to be known about each of them. In addition to being an important relationship system, totems were also an important contributor to the maintenance and management of knowledge.

Many things governed Aboriginal society, including totems. Totems can be animals, fish, trees, plants, reptiles, and all things in the landscape. People belonged to different totems. By the time they reached adulthood, every child understood their responsibilities and obligations to their totems and each other through the totemic system.

Being connected to living things in the environment through our totemic system enabled the individual to gain intimate knowledge of the totem they were connected to. For example, if you were connected to a certain type of tree, you would know if it was a medicine or a food or used for other things. You would know where it grew and how it grew.

If that tree grew in a certain type of soil, that tree would have a connection to the person whose totem was that certain type of soil. There is a relationship with all things around that tree, such as soil and the types of plants that grow in the vicinity. So there is a connection between all things.

This reflects a living community. Whether the area is a waterless area or a wet area, that ecosystem is a community. The people who have the totems of the things in that community also have obligations to one another and to that living community of nature, that totemic community.

In today's society, how well do we prepare young adults for the years ahead in terms of mind, body, and spirit? Do we leave it up to the school system or do we use our extended family to complement what the school is providing? Better still, do we create community learning cooperatives that schools, families, students, and others can participate in?

If a young adult faces an issue in their life, are they able to easily access support mechanisms that are culturally, socially, mentally, and emotionally safe? For many adolescents, the journey to young adulthood is far more difficult than it needs to be. In traditional times, the transition was one of flow supported by connected relationships. For a young person today, the transition is often one of dead ends and their progress is undermined by competitive isolation.

Young people are expected to compete for grades, compete for places in tertiary education, compete for jobs, compete for prominence on social media, and compete for attention. They live in a world where one must compete to be successful: a far cry from the Aboriginal world, where sharing is a cornerstone of community values and well-being.

In this modern-day world of competition, for every success, there are myriad rejections an individual has to overcome. Think about how many job applications have to be submitted before a person is successful (ten to fifteen per week is the suggested rate). Think about how many times actors, writers, musicians, entrepreneurs, sportspeople, and everyday people experience rejection in their lives. Rejection is a common, expected experience to the point where, as a society, we accept rejection as an almost noble part of the human condition.

Although resilience is an essential quality to have in our tool-box of life skills, a key to a life of well-being is maintaining balance in our lives. Too much rejection can create imbalance and lead to feelings of failure. Is this any way to treat our young people . . . or anyone, for that matter?

We can't accept everybody's job application, book manuscript, song, or business idea, of course, but we do need to think about better ways of supporting people's dreams and aspirations. Rather than closing a door, maybe we can help people find a corridor to another door that will open for them. By noticing what they have to offer and tapping into our networks, we can create a community of sharing rather than islands of rejection.

For most of us, there is a limit to the amount of rejection we can cope with. Once this point is crossed, we can give up trying. When this happens, our health is at great risk. This is a massive opportunity lost for all of our families, communities, towns, regions, states, countries, and the planet. It doesn't have to be this way, does it?

PARENT: As we transition from young adult to adult, our needs shift from establishing our identity and life purpose to that of living them. Our responsibilities increase as many of us seek a long-term partner and long-term security. In many instances we pursue these things as stepping stones to the goal of becoming a parent.

I have been blessed to be a new dad on three occasions. Being told by my wife, Alison, she was pregnant, feeling the baby kick, watching Alison's tummy grow, and witnessing the births of Rhys then Brianna then Liam are without a doubt the most precious experiences of my life. Now that I am a dad, I truly understand why Aboriginal spirituality regards women and motherhood so reverently.

When I first nursed each of our newborns, I felt indescribable love flow through every part of my being. After a few weeks of having them at home, my life became a contradiction of highs and lows as lack of sleep, seemingly unending crying, diaper changes, bottle feeds, washing, and managing the daily household routine became overwhelming at times.

In traditional Aboriginal society, these various challenges were mitigated by the ever-present support of extended family. The role of parenting was shared among the clan, with the baby having several mothers, fathers, and grandparents.

Everybody in an Aboriginal tribe was family and had obligations to each other in some way. Everybody had responsibility for everybody. Everything was shared in the day-to-day life of a tribal group.

The titles of father, mother, grandfather, grandmother, brother, and sister were used in a different way in traditional Aboriginal society. Under our skin system, a person who Western society would label a biological grandfather would have a number of other men connected to him through his "skin" connection. These men were seen as the child's grandfathers, too. So there is a much broader relationship and obligation among the tribe than two grandfathers to one grandchild.

One of the skin system's main roles was to ensure that people

who were closely related to each other didn't marry each
other. The old women oversaw this process. This was a serious
responsibility, and couples who tried to go around this system
were subjected to the most serious of punishments.

The benefits of community involvement in raising children
have been proven over tens of thousands of years in Aboriginal
society. These include:

- parents having time to do things that enhance their
  personal well-being;
- parents having time to do things that nurture their
  relationship;
- parents having time to carry out community-related
  responsibilities;
- the child having access to an increased diversity of
  experiences and learning;
- older people having a hands-on opportunity to participate
  in something important;
- older people having the hands-on opportunity to utilize
  their wealth of experience and learning in a productive
  way; and
- increased community connectivity, relationships, and
  networks.

Access to support in raising a child has always been important,
and is possibly even more important for parents in the world we
now live in. On the flip side, an inability to access support can
create stresses that negatively impact individual well-being and

undermine relationships to the detriment of parents, children, and society in general.

Creating local community support systems and networks for parents is therefore essential if we are to improve well-being at an individual, family, and community level.

ELDER: Many of us who are now in the autumn of our lives look back and reflect on how quickly time has passed. The children have grown up and left home and our needs might now relate to planning for retirement, coming to terms with what we have failed to achieve in our life, maintaining health, travel, social activities, and grandchildren.

For some, transitioning beyond middle age is an exciting proposition. For others, it can be a challenging time of loneliness and regret. In many communities there is an unfortunate disconnect between the elderly and the young.

In traditional times, Elders were of critical importance in ensuring the well-being of the community. In some ways, Elders had the largest portfolio of roles in the community, having responsibility for sharing story, song, or dance; teaching; leadership; governance; conflict resolution; and overseeing spiritual practice and ceremony.

An Elder was, and still is, a person who has accumulated knowledge and uses that knowledge in a positive way to lift a community.

Traditionally, the Elders had the knowledge of the stories and shared that knowledge with the young people as they earned the right to know these stories.

Before they died, the owner of the stories passed their stories on to the next generation.

In traditional Aboriginal society, the status of Elder was a highly respected one. To be given the status of Elder, an individual had to demonstrate over many years their understanding of and adherence to the Lore, including living the values of love, respect, humility, and sharing.

By the time an individual became an Elder, the Aboriginal system of lifelong learning (which integrated technical, academic, and spiritual knowledge) meant the Elders possessed a holistic toolbox of skills and wisdom that enabled them to be insightful, caring, pragmatic, forward-looking, strategic, and decisive in leadership.

Elders were therefore very connected to both the spirit world and the physical world in which they lived. This dual capability informed various high-level conversations on a range of topics relating to the well-being of the tribe and neighboring tribes—including marriages, trade, ceremonies, and environmental threats, such as drought and flood.

The Elders were the governing body when it came to making big decisions about what was going to happen. The decisions made were always for the good of the collective and in accordance with their responsibilities to their Country. The decision had to be unanimous rather than majority. Everybody had to agree and if one person disagreed, it would be discussed and discussed until everybody agreed.

Elders to this day are recognizable by their giving nature, their humility, and the air of serenity that surrounds them. Elders are often:

- comfortable with silence,
- quiet and reflective thinkers,
- patient,
- caring,
- firm (particularly with regard to enforcing values), and
- not prone to emotional outbursts.

They are often a rock for people who feel they are sinking in quicksand. Elders don't need to force themselves or their opinions onto anyone. They are ready and willing to help, but do not have a need to be seen or heard and do not strive for power.

Elders are still highly respected in the Aboriginal community. Their guidance is often sought on a range of matters and their advice highly valued. It is my observation and experience that this isn't so much the case with elderly people in the Western world. From an economic and social perspective, this is a sad and significant loss, given Elders and the elderly are a rich source of knowledge and wisdom for communities.

Have you got Elders or elderly people in your life? Is there an elderly person you have noticed in your community who you might like to talk to? Why don't you give them a smile, say hello, and ask them if they would mind a five-minute chat?

If you are able to build a relationship with them, there will be the opportunity to learn about each other . . . to hear each other's stories. We don't do enough of this in our life. Everyone has a story and everyone's story has wisdom, inspiration and learning embedded in it. Most people are reluctant to share their stories as they think they are unremarkable, yet we are all remarkable. So go ahead, give an older person a chance to realize this. In doing so, you just don't know what you both might learn.

People in their elderly years can still be a significant and positive force. They may not be able to run as fast or jump as high as they used to, but this is balanced by their increased experience and wisdom, which can enable them to contribute to numerous relationships in a rich and unique way.

We owe it to ourselves, our children, and our communities to connect with this most valuable resource.

VERY OLD: As we start to approach the end of our story, the last years of our life, our physical capability and energy levels are probably not as substantial as they once were. When we become very old, our needs may be focused on giving back to those who are important to us and accepting the life we have lived.

For far too many very old people, social isolation and loneliness can become the norm . . . to the point where they can start to feel they have been forgotten and that their story is unimportant. At a time of life when relationships can become scarce, strong and caring connections become more important than ever.

In traditional times, most Aboriginal people lived to be very old (unlike today, when the life expectancy of an Aboriginal person is much lower than that of a non-Aboriginal person). There were many reasons for this:

- healthy diet,
- regular exercise (walking Country),
- systems to support good mental health practice,
- embedded spiritual practice in daily life,

- an ongoing involvement with community and related sense of purpose,
- a pharmacy of bush medicines that could address most sicknesses that arose,
- multiple active relationships that mitigated loneliness and isolation, and
- continued care from the entire community.

The very old were looked after in all aspects of their life, given they were the most highly regarded people in the tribe. Although the very old were not as active as they once were, they could still be involved in Elders' discussions if they chose to or were asked to.

These Old People lived a little bit apart from the rest of the community and were revered for their sacred knowledge. It was a privilege to sit with them and hear that knowledge being imparted.

As I grew up, I saw the Old People a lot. I learned to respect them because of their positive actions in teaching me about Country. I learned to respect all things in Country because all things in Country gave something back, and if I sang for it and danced for it and I held stories in my heart, it was always there for me.

There was never a need for my Elders to demand respect. It was given because of their positive actions, their caring, and sharing for all things as equals.

How do we treat our very old in society today? Are they highly respected, revered, and supported? Do you regularly connect with very old people?

Very old people can be entertaining and uplifting. Elder-care facilities are delightful places to visit. Within their walls are the most special resources in our community. For those who are younger (say twenty to forty years of age), the elderly can become highly valued surrogate grandparents, uncles, and aunts. In return, the younger people can become highly valued surrogate grandchildren, nephews, and nieces. Many lives would benefit from these kinds of relationships.

Sometimes you might meet an old person who seems to be overly angry or negative. If you ever meet someone who is like this, why not see this as a wonderful opportunity to hear their story, understand why they feel the way they do, and perhaps help them find more joy in life.

If we think about our community as a tree, and then think about all the different parts that make up a tree, we see each part has a purpose and a role to play. Even when the leaves fall to the ground and they seem dead, they are still playing a part in the survival of that tree.

When our Old People pass away, their story stays with us if we remember it and if their story was strong. As we remember and tell their story, they are still contributing to our society.

They are like the leaves that fall from the tree. Even though the leaves are dead, they are still contributing to the life of that tree. If you rake those leaves away from the tree and burn them, that leaf can no longer contribute or play its role.

So if you take the stories of the Old People away, they can't play their roles—and this is why we must keep telling their stories. We should strive to be like the people we remember. Leave a good story for others to follow.

As you think about the importance of relationships and reflect on the Aboriginal life cycle I have just described to you, try to embrace the Aboriginal view of family. As you do this, you might find you have a broadened understanding of the relationships you could create to support your well-being journey and the well-being journeys of others.

Family was bigger than blood and biological connection. Aboriginal families, even if not blood related, through the kinship system were still related as if they were blood relatives. Everybody in a whole group or Nation was related to each other in some way and had kinship obligations and responsibilities to one another and to all things as the kinship system extended beyond humans.

It extended to the stars, plants, rocks, mountains, animals, and birds. The kinship system included everything. If you wanted to walk from one side of Australia to another, all the way through that Country you would have kinship obligations and family responsibilities, and through these responsibilities you had connection with that Country.

Exercise: Relationships

Reflect on the relationships you currently have in each grouping below. If it helps, rate yourself out of five for each category: one meaning you don't have any relationships and five meaning you have fantastic relationships in that category. Are there any categories that are important to you that you need to work on?

- Children
- Young people
- Young adults
- Parents
- Grandparents/the elderly
- Very old
- Work colleagues
- Social contacts
- Sporting contacts
- Other

Regardless of whether you are a baby, child, young adult, new parent, elderly, or very old person, personal relationships are a critical component of your well-being. It is therefore important to invest your time in creating and nurturing them. It is also important to think about your relationship with the land.

The way we live puts huge pressure on our environment. To feed population and economic growth, we destroy forests, we destroy rivers, and we dig big holes in the ground. Where do the creatures go when the forests are taken away? Where do the forest people live when the forests are taken away? The truth is, they don't. They become extinct.

We need to acknowledge that the way we live eradicates the existence of other people, animals, and plants. These special relationships have been betrayed. If we don't acknowledge this, we will never address it.

So I am not just asking big corporations to think about it.

I am asking every individual to think about it. And then after you think about it, I am asking you to do something about it. Because if you don't, who will?

Future generations of people, plants, animals, fish, trees, insects, and so on won't exist if we don't do something. The system that has destroyed the forests and the rivers and has made so many living things extinct will one day reach your doorstep and you might be the next thing facing extinction.

Not that long ago, many people would have scoffed at any reference to human extinction. Our recent experience of global pandemic has challenged that view. This, combined with the specter of the climate crisis, is a timely reminder of our fragility, our planet's fragility, and our need to respect our obligations and responsibilities to care for our place and all things in our place. We cannot do this without establishing the right relationships.

The more relationships we can create, the more story we can share. The more story we can share, the more knowledge we can pass on. The more knowledge we can pass on, the more informed discussion we can have on things that are mutually important. The more discussion we can have on things that are mutually important, the more we can agree on what needs to be done. The more we can agree on what needs to be done, the closer we are to a united vision. The closer we are to a united vision, the more effective we will be at making the changes needed for a better world.

The process outlined above is not new. For tens of thousands of years, Aboriginal people have gathered to reinforce relationships, share knowledge, discuss priorities, agree on actions, and make changes that ensure the well-being of all. Gatherings held in southeastern Queensland when the bunya nut was ready for harvest and in the Australian Alps when the bogong moth migrated are well-known examples of events at which tribal groups gathered to share food, conduct ceremonies, trade materials, arrange marriages, and discuss issues of Lore.

In the old traditional times before the Lore was taken away, we had stories that went right across Australia. These big Lore stories were of ancestors like the goanna who traveled Country, the echidna who traveled Country, and the rainbow snake who traveled through Country making rivers and creeks. That snake was very knowledgeable. He taught us the rules.

We all had these stories about these animals and even though these stories might have been a little different in different places, they also had a lot of similarities. That is what gave us connection to one another.

People from different tribes traveled right across the continent following these big storylines and meeting up with other people who were walking along the same tracks, listening, looking, sharing, dancing, singing, and doing ceremony together.

There were more than five hundred different Aboriginal languages in Australia when the boats first came. Maybe there are more than fifteen hundred dialects of those languages, and according to the latest science we have been here for more than 200,000 years. Think about it. We have been here for more than 200,000 years and we still had five hundred language groups and fifteen hundred dialects.

We lived on a big island. If we hadn't had the same big story, if we hadn't had the same respect, the same protocols, if we hadn't had unity, one Aboriginal Nation or an alliance of Aboriginal Nations could have formed and conquered all the other Nations, and we would have been speaking one language—like the British Empire tried to force peoples all over the world to do, like the Roman Empire tried to do, like the Greek Empire tried to do. They went out to try to conquer the world. They are called great civilizations, but what is so great about what they did? They stole, they killed, they destroyed, and they controlled. Our people didn't try to go out to conquer anyone because they had one Lore that gave them respect for one another.

That's why when you look at how Aboriginal people lived before 1788, you won't find one castle. If you go to Europe, there are castles everywhere. You will see castles in Ireland, Scotland, France, and other places in Europe—because in these places, people for thousands and thousands of years were frightened to lie down and go to sleep because of the wars and threats that surrounded them.

But in Australia, we never had the need for a castle; we never had one fort. People say, "Aah, that's because you blackfullas didn't know how to build one." No . . . it's not because we couldn't build one. If you go to a place in central western New South Wales called Brewarrina, there are stone walls built in the river that are three to four feet of rock work to catch fish. Those rocks have been there for more than 35,000 years: they are 30,000 years older than the Egyptian pyramids. They are built strong and have survived flood after flood and still work.

So we had the ability to build a castle—we just didn't have the need to build a castle.

We never built weapons of war. You won't find one place where there are masses of Aboriginal burials of our people dying by the spear. We built tools or weapons to hunt and gather because that is the way we lived. But we only ever took what we needed. We had unity right across the land. There were fights between individuals but it never translated into tribal warfare because of the ceremonial connections between us.

In traditional times, everyone was part of one Lore. Everybody had Lore and everybody had respect for one another. So when the first fleet arrived in Australia, the Aboriginal people would have most likely thought, "These people have come to visit us. They will have the Lore like everybody else does. They will share with us, they will do ceremony with us. We will feed them and we will have a good time together. Then they will go back home and leave us with good stories that we can share."

But that didn't happen. The boat people came and they didn't have the same values or Lore that Aboriginal people had and they started to destroy the landscape. Because the landscape was full of spirit and alive, when the boat people started to cut up rocks and build sandstone dwellings, they were killing ancestors, because some of the people were related to stone and rocks. When they started to cut down trees, they were killing some people's ancestors, because some people were related to trees. And so things happened that created a lot of bad feeling between Black and white people in Australia.

So our Lore, Aboriginal Lore, once upon a time was shared with all. It is time to do this once again.

It could be argued that the world has never been so connected. Advances in computer, satellite, and communications technology have reshaped the way we communicate (via multiple devices and media), the speed at which information is shared (almost instant), and the growth of knowledge (doubling every thirteen months).

This technological advancement has not yet translated at an international level into the advancement of relationships or the unity, goodwill, and spirit of sharing that good relationships foster. Rather than improved unity, we are still seeing division, suspicion, and insularity.

If you look at how people in the Western world go about their daily lives, in many cases it is very much opposite to the way Aboriginal people live. For most, the day is made up of discrete modules of activity, such as eating, work, study, leisure, exercise, and chores. Although most of these activities might involve interaction with other people, often not enough time is provided to develop and nurture meaningful relationships.

Modern life is often a solo race against the clock as we try to get everything ticked off our "to do" lists so we can get on top of things in readiness for the next day, when we restart the same cycle. People rarely talk to strangers, and homes are fortresses with locks, bars, and fences. Our biological wiring to socialize is being corroded by a lifestyle of alienation, isolation, and solitude as we understandably seek refuge from the busyness that envelops us.

In traditional times, food gathering, eating, caring for community, caring for place, learning, playing, socializing, exercising, and nurturing relationships were integrated activities underpinned by spiritual beliefs and cultural values that meant every minute of life had purpose and meaning.

Rather than being a series of events with start and end points, traditional life was a flow of integrated activities where time had limited relevance. There was no such thing as a stranger, given that everybody was kin in one way or another, and housing structures facilitated communal communication and integration. Socialization within the family, extended family, clan, tribe, neighboring tribes, and across the continent was of paramount importance in upholding the Lore.

The Western world could benefit from the traditional Aboriginal way of people making more time to connect with each other and building relationships across the demographic spectrum. The more relationships we build, the more connected we become. The more we connect, the more we share.

In traditional Aboriginal society, everything was based on sharing. Not just giving, not just taking, but sharing.

The journey of the ancestors was about putting things into Country and sometimes taking things from Country. By giving and receiving without keeping score, you are sharing.

When you share with one another it shows you care for one another.

Is the journey you are on about you and what you want or is it, like the journeys of the ancestors, about sharing? Is it about giving sometimes, receiving sometimes and sharing with the people who are on the same journey as you? Or is your journey about the "selfish you," where you don't think about others?

Will you share what you have with others so people around you can become sharers also? By doing this, we all become carers. Have you got others walking with you or have you discarded them? When you look back, do you see one track or many tracks alongside yours?

For most of us, the initial stages of the COVID-19 pandemic involved mandatory isolation in our homes. Many people found the inability to meet with loved ones, to go outside and connect with nature, or to attend group gatherings a very difficult experience that placed emotional and mental health at risk. Although technology provided a welcome link to loved ones, it wasn't quite the same.

As lockdown requirements were lifted and before health experts raised fears of a second wave of COVID-19, people joyfully embraced their newfound freedom and the opportunity to reconnect with other people, with Country, with social activities, and with recreational pursuits. It is often the case we don't appreciate what we have until it is gone. Being able to sit with our beloved people is a privilege we need to acknowledge and give thanks for, long after COVID-19 becomes a distant memory.

During the worst of the crisis, we watched our televisions in fear as the stark statistics reminded us of our mortality. At the same time, we saw inspiring acts of courage, sharing, and caring (health workers, supermarket workers, other essential workers), and uplifting video footage of unity (Italian people singing from balconies, virtual concerts) that reminded us of the power of connection.

Through any crisis, there are powerful lessons to be learned and not forgotten. Let's hope that the importance of relationships is one of those!

Message 3

It is vital for each of us to create, nurture, and sustain relationships, including with the land, babies, children, young people, young adults, adults, parents, Elders, and the very old.

Message 4

Our celebration of diversity must be underpinned by a platform of unity.

Message 5

Always share.

Chapter 3

Love, Gratitude, and Humility

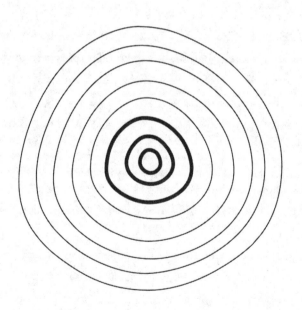

Way back in the Ngurrampaa, in the beginning of time, the echidna, or thikarbilla, had no spikes on his back. He was just a little furry animal like a rabbit. There was this old man who loved to eat the thikarbilla.

One day, he got his two grandsons and he said, "Boys, we are going hunting for thikarbilla. Listen to me. You know I am your grandfather and you have to come and do what you are told because that's the Lore."

And the two boys said, "But Grandfather, you also have an obligation to us. When we get thikarbilla you are supposed to share it with us, but everywhere we go you are too greedy and eat it on your own."

And the grandfather said, "Well . . . I will share this time. Come with me."

And so they went out hunting, looking for thikarbilla, and the old man got tired because he was fat and got tired easily. And so he sat on the ground and said, "You two boys. You go and look for thikarbilla."

And the boys went out and found a thikarbilla and brought it back to their grandfather. He said, "Leave that thikarbilla here with me and you go and get some wood." They went and got some wood and brought it back to their grandfather and he said, "That's not enough wood. Go and get some more." So the boys went away to get more wood, and while they were away, that old man lit a fire, cooked up the thikarbilla, and he ate it.

When the boys came back, they asked their grandfather, "Where is that thikarbilla?"

He replied, "Well . . . you took too long. I got too hungry."

The boys asked, "Where's ours?" and the grandfather said, "You will have to go and get another one. Go and get another one."

The boys went out and found another one, and while they were away the old man got the wood that they had brought back the second time and hid it behind his back. And when they returned, they put the thikarbilla down and he said, "Oh . . . there is no wood left. I had to burn it all because you took too long. You had better go get some more wood. Leave that thikarbilla with me and go get some more wood."

The boys put the thikarbilla down and went off to get more wood, and while they were gone, the old man got the wood out from behind his back and he cooked that thikarbilla up and ate it. And this went on and on. And the old man got fatter and fatter. And the two boys started to get really, really hungry because the old man wouldn't share with them.

Back in the days of the Ngurrampaa, at the beginning of time, butterflies were magic. And they flew by and they saw the old man and they saw what he was doing wrong. And they said, "That old man is breaking the Lore. Instead of being loving and thankful, he is being greedy. Instead of being humble, he is being a bully. He's not sharing and he's not fulfilling his obligation to the Lore. He isn't looking after those boys as he should. They are looking after him but he's not looking after them." The butterflies fluttered their wings in anger. "Let's go back to our tree," they said.

There was a tree the butterflies belonged to called a waria bush. On the waria bush were lots of sharp sticks. The butterflies went back to their tree and collected many of these sharp sticks. By this time, the old man had eaten so many thikarbilla he was starting to look like one. The butterflies came back to the old man, and because he had broken the Lore, and because he was starting to look like a thikarbilla, they decided they were going to turn him into one. And so they turned him into a thikarbilla. And then they speared him with all their sharp sticks for not fulfilling his obligation to the boys. And that's how the thikarbilla got its spikes.

When the boys came back the butterflies said, "Boys. Look at what your grandfather has become. He is a thikarbilla. He has been speared and he's got spikes all over his back because he has broken the Lore. And that is what happens to people who break the Lore. They get speared.

"But don't you worry, you two boys. We will care for you. You can go back to our tree . . . our tree where we sleep and live. On that tree there is fruit. And that fruit is there for you kids. Only kids are allowed to go and get that fruit. No adults can ever have it."

Most of us would agree that love is a basic necessity in our life. Through the centuries there have been numerous descriptions of love, including romantic, affectionate, self, familial, unconditional, enduring, playful, unrequited, empty, consummate, and infatuated. Is it any wonder love can be such a confusing experience to navigate?

Despite the difficulty in trying to describe what love is, in simple terms, love can be thought of as a complex set of emotions, behaviors, and beliefs associated with strong feelings of affection, protectiveness, warmth, and respect for a person, thing, or practice. So it is something we feel.

After learning a lot of stories, you learn to love your place because it gives you everything you need. Love is a really important part of Aboriginal society.

In some religions, they say humans are sinners born into a world of sin. That is not our way. We believe we are conceived in love and born in love.

We are born into a world of love and are surrounded by love all of our lives, including love from our family, love from our Country, and love from our Spirit Ancestors. When we die, we leave in love and go back to love. Love is all around us.

Aboriginal spirituality is anchored in love. The creation story told at the start of Chapter 1 reflects the love of the Mother and the Father. Their love led to the Mother becoming pregnant and the birth of all things, including us. We were conceived from love and born of love.

There are thousands of stories about the Father across the continent. Some of these stories describe how he lives in the sky watching over us, loving us, and wanting us to live a good story. Traditional stories in my Country describe how the Father comes to earth in human form to visit his people and teach us how to love and care for each other and everything around us. At numerous sacred sites in my Country, there are footprints in stone that are tens of thousands of years old. These are the Father's footprints. They show us where he once stood and taught us the Lore.

About eighty miles inland of the New South Wales Central Coast there is a very important mountain called Mount Yengo. This mountain is a very important part of our belief system. In the beginning, this flat-top mountain was a real living animal called the echidna. In my language she is called Thikarbilla. Like many other creation animals, she was traveling through Country making different landscapes according to what Biamii, the Father, had asked her to do.

Along the journey, children were born to her. These children fell asleep and became smaller mountains in the landscape. When the mother thikarbilla rested, she fell asleep also and became Mount Yengo. In the beginning, Mount Yengo was much higher and rounder than it is today. It was shaped just like an echidna.

One day, after spending time in Country teaching his people the Lore, it was time for Biamii to return to his home. When Biamii, our sky father, saw how high Thikarbilla was, he used her to step up into the sky. This is why the mountain now has a flat top. From that time onward, whenever Biamii ascended to the sky in this Country, he always stepped from Mount Yengo. It became the stepping place of God.

Many of the rock carvings found in the region of Mount Yengo were put there by Biamii to teach us the Lore.

Mount Yengo is only one of many stories of journeys of our animal ancestors who traveled across Australia and connected us to one another.

No matter what I do in this life, no matter what disappointments and sadness I may face in interpersonal love, I know I am always loved by the Father.

Although the Father's love for the Mother is infinite, he can't be with her as he would like. His responsibilities require him to be in the sky. He sacrifices his love for the Mother so he can uphold his love for us.

The Mother is so beautiful that when we pass over to the spirit world, once rested, our spirit may choose to come back to Country to continue caring for the Mother and all things on her. Just like a human mother, the Mother loves all her children, whether they be mammals, reptiles, birds, fish, insects, or humans. She wants them all to live a good story. But just like a human mother, the Mother knows she needs to let her children make choices and mistakes so they can learn and grow. Her love is so selfless that she still loves her children even when they hurt her.

People who still believe in the old ways feel extreme sadness when they see land being destroyed, the rivers being dammed, the trees cut down, and the ground being dug up. It is no different to them than if you were to come home to your mother's house and find her being raped, stabbed, and mutilated. How you would feel is how the Old People feel when they see the Mother, the land, suffering the same pain and humiliation.

The Old People tell us that the human race needs the Mother more than she needs us. As we continue to hurt her, the Mother cries for us. Her love is unconditional, but she despairs at how we have lost our way. A cornerstone of the Lore is responsibility. As a collective, human beings are breaking the Lore on a global scale. In our spirituality, this means there will be consequences. First there will be warnings . . . and then there will be punishment.

The Spirit Ancestors exist everywhere across our Country. The changes forced upon the landscape over the past two hundred and thirty years, including the establishment of cities, towns, fences, mines, and dams, have not driven the Spirit Ancestors away. In places where there is still story, song, and dance, the spirits are active. In other places, they are waiting. Waiting for the time when the stories are shared once again, when voices sing for them once again, when people dance for them once again. They are watching, waiting for the time when the right people are ready to listen.

In thinking about the concept of love, it is important to not think about it as an isolated practice. Love cannot be fully understood and shared without understanding the importance of the Lore and the responsibilities we have to follow the Lore.

In our way, love should always follow Lore. Now, a lot of people from other religions say to me, "I think you have got it wrong. I think love should be first," and I say to them, "There have been many destructive things done around the world under the banner of love. People have gone out into the world thinking other people needed their love and instead of making the world better they have destroyed some good things."

That's basically what happened to Aboriginal people after

the boats arrived. People thought we needed their help, guidance, and insights, and people thought we needed their society and we needed their rules. They might have come with love but they didn't know our story.

The first thing we have to know before we can help anybody is their story. We have to know the Lore relating to their story; that is, we have to know the rules, responsibilities, and obligations relating to their story. Once we know their story, then we can act in love because we will respect their story and make sure what we do fits in with that story. What we do will be right.

But if we don't know their story, we aren't really acting with love because love includes respect, tolerance, acceptance, and understanding. If we don't know their story, we can do more harm to them than good.

The love of the Father, the Mother, and the Spirit Ancestors is there for any of us willing to learn about the Lore and uphold the associated responsibilities. You may have already had a small taste of this love. Any time you sit in nature, be still and feel joy and peace flow through you, you are connecting with the love of the Mother.

Exercise: Connecting with Place 3

The aim of this exercise is to help you connect with place. It might help if you record the words so you can listen to them with your eyes closed or perhaps have someone read the script to you.

Find a comfortable place outside where you can connect with nature. It could be in your yard if you have one. It could be somewhere close by that you connect to or it could be a very special place away from any sign of human impact.

Find a place to sit in comfort.

Let the chatter of your mind slip into the background. There are always things to think about in the now, but for the moment, you can let it all disappear.

With all the time in the world, look around you. What can you see? What can you hear?

Now close your eyes and focus on the ground below you. Notice how your bare feet are connected to the ground and how good it feels. Notice how the way you are seated feels so strong and connected to the earth that nothing could knock you over.

When you are ready, imagine gathering a ball of light around your navel. This energy represents your love and thanks for everything the Mother gives you. Let it build and build . . . feel how joyous the light is in your belly.

When it feels right, send this light in a gentle stream down through you into the ground with as much love as you can summon. Let it flow and flow deeper and deeper. Let it flow into the center of the earth.

When you have emptied your belly of the light, give thanks to the earth and all the things the earth gives you that keep you alive . . . food, oxygen, water, shelter . . . all these things are from the Mother.

When the time feels right, imagine an energy beam coming from the center of the earth. This energy is solely for you; no one else. This is a time for you; no one else. You are worthy of this time . . . so relax and enjoy it.

Imagine the light gently coming up from the earth, through you into your navel region. As it builds, feel the joy and feel the peace creating a warm glow right across your midsection.

Let the ball of energy flow gently through your entire body . . . notice what you are feeling . . . you might feel a tingling sensation . . . you might feel contentment . . . you might feel other things . . . you might not feel anything at all. If you don't feel anything, there is no need to worry . . . just trust that this energy is real and that it is there for you.

When you are ready . . . gently and in no particular rush . . . let the connection go and, in your own time, come back to the now.

How do you feel? How did you feel during the exercise? If you felt a sense of peace, or perhaps joy, or perhaps love, or perhaps all of these things, you have connected with the love of the Mother. If you haven't felt a sense of peace, that's OK. Keep on carrying out the exercise without pressuring yourself to achieve any particular outcome. You might be making great progress but just not feeling it, so trust the process and try to let go of the destination. It took me a while to totally connect, but it was a great investment.

If you felt something during the above exercise: well done. This experience is something you can build on. Because of the many years I have been practicing my connection to the love of the Father, the Mother, and the Spirit Ancestors, I am able to tap into this unlimited source of love whenever I feel the need. My faith and belief have carried me through some very difficult times.

Beliefs relating to the Father, the Mother, and the Spirit Ancestors have given Aboriginal people strength and guidance for a very long time.

Uncle Paul and I don't expect you to believe what we believe . . .

but we expect you to respect what we believe . . . as we respect what you believe. Spirituality isn't a competition where there is only one winner. There is much to be shared and there is much to be learned between us. The important thing is we have a connection to something bigger than ourselves in a way that gives us meaning for life, death, and the nature of reality. This kind of connection can be seen as a kind of spiritual love.

If you are reading this book and don't really believe in spiritual love, then you are going to find it hard to connect with or believe in the love of the Father, the Mother, or the Spirit Ancestors, which is completely OK. There is still a great deal of information in it that will be very useful to you.

In Aboriginal culture, spiritual love is critical to our well-being but it does not stand alone. Impersonal love (our love for an object, principle, or goal) and interpersonal love (love between human beings) are types of love that are also critical for us to live a good story.

In terms of impersonal love, I have strong affection and warmth for travel, food, walking Country, sport, movies, writing, and hot baths. I could add more, of course, but I suspect I have given an insight into how many things I love. Uncle Paul loves living on his remote property away from the hustle and bustle, walking Country, campfire cooking, sharing culture, solar energy, motorcars, and dark chocolate (if you ever want his instant attention, dark chocolate is the key).

In our personal relationships, it is important to let those we love know how special they are to us. If we don't communicate our feelings, they might never know how special they are. Uncle Paul and I are fortunate to be able to mentor a large group of men.

If you ever see us when we catch up with each other, you will notice we have no embarrassment about expressing our love with a first-up hug, regardless of where we are (in shopping centers, on busy main streets, and in parking lots, we often extract confused glances from onlookers). We also have no problem saying that we love each other—verbally or when we text each other.

Imagine how great it would be if there was more of this happening in the broader community? The more we express our love, the more space we create for loving acts to grow. The more love grows, the more sharing takes place. The more sharing takes place, the more caring becomes the norm. The more caring becomes the norm, the more goodwill spreads. The more goodwill spreads, the greater the likelihood for the world to become a better place.

Interpersonal love is part of our nature. We might love our family members, friends, and partners but find it hard to say it. Now is the perfect time to challenge yourself.

Interpersonal love can be a difficult experience to navigate, particularly with regards to romantic love. The internal and external pressures to find romantic love that start in our teenage years will invariably lead to some form of heartbreak for most of us, given that up to 70 percent of relationships break up in the first year. When our heart is broken, it is important to allow healing to occur over whatever time is needed to ensure the scarring doesn't undermine our ability to love in the future.

Separately from the devastating experience of heartbreak, sometimes people can become so infatuated—whether it be by a material thing or a person—that they become preoccupied with a fear of losing that thing or person. Instead of feeling joyful, they can find themselves entrenched in a cycle of anxiety.

The Lore teaches us that all things are transient, so rather than worry about what we have lost or the possibility of losing what we have, enjoy the moment. In traditional times, part of daily life was giving thanks and love on a continual basis for everything that was given to us—food, shelter, forest, animals, the sky, and relationships.

Although the many gifts given to us by the Father, the Mother, and the Spirit Ancestors are there for us to enjoy, it is important that we don't overindulge. The Lore tells us we must never be greedy and we must never take something for ourselves if it disrespects or takes away from another. The Lore also teaches us we must never steal.

Sometimes we have different stories about the same thing. This is another story about the echidna.

Thikarbilla was hungry. He poked his nose here, he poked his nose there. He was smaller than a newborn baby, with a thick coating of hair that protected him from insect bites, which was handy given how much he loved insects. Every now and then he found a morsel of food that he quickly devoured, but no matter how many things he ate, he was still hungry.

He had just wiped his nose clean of some dirt from an ants' nest when he smelled something that made him close his eyes and smile. It was the smell of a freshly cooked kangaroo, and Thikarbilla knew he just had to find where the smell was coming from.

He moved as quickly as his little legs could carry him, up small hills, down small hills, across a dry creek bed, and through some long grass until finally there it was. Thikarbilla could see, lying on a tree branch out of reach of most animals, a freshly cooked kangaroo.

He looked left, he looked right, and then he turned around in a circle to see who might have placed the kangaroo there. He couldn't see any people, but he could see many footprints heading toward the river.

"Aah," he said to himself. "This mob has cooked that kangaroo and placed it in the tree to cool while they go and gather vegetables by the river." He walked to the edge of the hill that went down to the river and could see the people gathering food, talking, and laughing in the distance.

Good, *he thought as he scuttled back to the tree and climbed it.* I am so hungry. This is just what I need, *he thought as he pushed the cooked kangaroo out of the tree and dragged it next to the campfire, which was still burning.*

As he took the first bite, Thikarbilla groaned with pleasure. "This is the best thing I have ever eaten," he said out loud before taking another bite and another and another. Thikarbilla was enjoying his tucker so much that he forgot about the people down by the river. Soon he had eaten so much that he could hardly move but that didn't stop him from eating. I am so hungry, *he thought as he continued to eat.*

"Hey. Look. There's a thikarbilla and he's eating our kangaroo!" a woman screamed. "He's a thief."

Thikarbilla's full belly wobbled this way and that as he slowly turned around and saw an old woman shaking a digging stick at him and looking very angry.

"Naaah. You got it all wrong," Thikarbilla said in his most

cheerful voice. "I could see you all down at the river gathering your vegetables and I thought I would get that kangaroo down from the tree and put it near the fire so you could eat it as soon as you got back."

The old woman took a step closer. She shook her digging stick at him and looked even more angry. "Not only is he a thief, this thikarbilla is a liar," the old woman yelled. "He's broken the Lore." She looked over at a number of younger men. "He's broken the Lore. You fullas . . . go and spear him."

So the young men speared Thikarbilla, but still he kept on talking, repeating his story over and over again.

"He's not even saying he's done the wrong thing. He's refusing to tell the truth. Spear him some more," the old woman said.

The young men speared Thikarbilla again and again until his entire body from front to back was covered in spears . . . but still he kept on lying.

"Here. He still won't shut up," the old woman said. "Spear him in the head. That should stop it."

The young men speared Thikarbilla in the head, but still he kept on denying having done anything wrong.

"Ay . . . he's talking out his backside. Spear him there. That will shut him up."

The young men speared Thikarbilla in the bottom and finally he shut up.

Because he was a thief and a liar, the many spears on Thikarbilla are with him to this day as a reminder to all things to not be greedy and to always tell the truth.

My grandmother used to love telling me that story. And when

she did, she used to laugh at the end of it and say, "See, Pauly, there are a lot of people like him. They talk and talk out of their backsides, thinking that we believe them."

The Lore tells us how much we are loved and that we must love all that is around us. The Lore also tells us our love needs to be demonstrated through our actions.

Exercise: Practicing Love

Listed below are a number of ways that we can demonstrate love for ourselves and others through our actions. For each of these actions, rate yourself from one to five. A rating of one means you are terrible at the action; a rating of five means you excel.

- I am kind to others.
- I am kind to myself.
- I accept people for what they are and do not judge.
- I accept myself and love myself (warts and all).
- I aim to create unity in whatever I do, rather than division.
- I tell those I care about that I love them.
- I regularly help others.
- I care very much for the earth and all things on the earth.
- I am good at sharing (time, knowledge, goodwill, material things).
- I nurture others.
- I nurture myself.

Any actions where you have rated yourself a one or two require urgent reflection on changes you might choose to make in your life. A rating of three is an area to consider as possibly needing improvement also.

In essence, the chapters of this book reflect how to practice a loving approach to life. If we care for our place; build and nurture a diversity of relationships; share what we have; promote unity; practice continuous gratitude; act in a humble way; commit to lifelong learning; be truthful; inspire others; live in the moment; heal from our past; seek contentment; and lead others in an authentic way, we honor the love we are conceived through and born into. By accepting the love that surrounds us and by redistributing that love to other people and other things, we are more able to fulfill the responsibilities of the Lore, follow the Dreaming Path, and achieve a state of well-being.

Throughout the world, we see examples of love in practice that move us to the point of tears. During the recent bushfires in Australia and forest fires in the American West, firefighters, some of whom had seen their own houses burn to the ground, stayed on duty tirelessly to protect others from the same fate. During the global pandemic, health workers placed themselves in great danger to sustain the lives of others. In both instances, lives were lost. There is no greater testimony of love. We need to reflect on what these heroes stood for and learn from their selflessness. We need to use their stories to unite us.

Their stories should never be forgotten. They remind us of the remarkable power of love and hopefully encourage each of us to be more caring, to be more loving, and to have gratitude for what we have right here right now.

Even though most of us are deeply moved when we hear of the inspiring selfless acts of others, how often do we convert that feeling into action? How do you think we rate as a collective in terms of demonstrating loving practice in our daily life?

On any given day there are numerous opportunities to share goodwill and kindness with others but how often do we see this happening? We can choose to share goodwill or kindness with a neighbor or with a stranger. We can do this while walking down the street, driving in traffic, traveling on public transport, wandering through a shopping center, at work, or even in our lounge room at home.

We can also share goodwill and kindness with people we might never meet in person through taking the time to understand what others might be going through and even joining online petition groups or funding efforts. Every day gives us countless opportunities to be kind and to be thankful for what we have compared to others.

When an Australian writer-performer asked for donations to support Australian bushfire relief, people from all over the world answered the call with donations totaling $51 million Australian. This is overwhelming evidence of the platform of goodwill and kindness that already exists in the world. It is gratifying to know that the opportunity to grow love across the world is not coming from a zero base.

Finding the positive around us makes it much easier to practice love. Although there are always things that can bring us down, focusing on the negative can be an addictive and unhealthy experience. This doesn't mean we ignore problems that we face, but it does mean we don't allow the gray cloak of despair to cover the color that surrounds us in abundance. A good way to harvest the positive in every day is to adopt a mindset of thankfulness.

We might not see them until we look, but there are lots of things in our lives to be thankful for. A good starting point is giving thanks for being alive, since the odds of a human being born are 1 in 6×10^{100}. That is, your chance of having been born is:

1 in 60,000,000,000,000,000,000,000,000,000,000,000,000,000,000, 000,000,000,000,000,000,000,000,000,000,000,000,000,000,000,000, 000,000,000.

The fact you are even here is therefore a miracle!

In Aboriginal spirituality, conception is not a random biological miracle at all. Conception is the result of a sacred connection that provides the opportunity for a soul to reenter the world from the Spirit Pool. The soul reenters the world for a purpose. You are here for a purpose. It is good to remember this in times of doubt, when you might be feeling lost and beginning to ask yourself, "What's the point?"

When we find ourselves wondering this, rather than worrying about the future we can choose to connect to the now. We can start to identify what we can be thankful for. If we do this in a humble way, we might begin to realize we have much to feel good about. Perhaps you are grateful for some of these benefits:

- a roof over your head
- people who care about you
- no major health problems
- parks and gardens you can visit
- libraries where you can access knowledge or books
- bushland to sit in

- mountain ranges to admire from afar
- clouds idly floating by, continually shape-shifting
- the sun's rays
- a breeze on a warm day that makes you feel alive
- a breeze on a cold day that makes you feel alive
- the smell of freshly brewed coffee
- chocolate, ice cream, or other things to spoil yourself with occasionally
- music to listen to or sing to loudly in the car or shower
- hot water
- laughter

The opportunities are endless. When we express gratitude, it lifts us and gives us the ability to energize and lift others who might not be feeling so great.

Feeling thankful can be difficult when the ongoing pressures of living wear us down and life is a chore. Daily activities such as working, packing children's lunches, washing up dishes, doing laundry, shopping, cooking, and cleaning can feel like unpleasant and draining impositions on our freedom. Rather than pinning our hopes of fixing the problem on winning the lottery (long odds), we can remedy the situation by reshaping the way we think (very good odds).

For traditional Aboriginal society, nothing in life was a chore because all tasks were infused with spirituality. All tasks were carried out with respect, with thankfulness, and with gratitude.

When a task feels like a chore, it is because we are thinking of the task as a chore rather than seeing it as an opportunity to practice goodwill and love.

- When you are working (you are also generating income to pay the bills).
- When you are packing lunches for your children (you are also caring for them and saving money).
- When you are washing up dishes (you are also giving someone else the time to do something else).
- When you are shopping for groceries (you are also accessing things you need to live).
- When you are cooking (you are also providing nurture for your body).
- When you are cleaning (you are maintaining a healthy living environment).

These are all things to give thanks for rather than chores. It is all about changing the way you view the world. If you see life as a never-ending uphill battle, that is what your lived experience will be.

Exercise: Gratitude Diary

Find a blank notepad, exercise book, or journal. It doesn't have to be fancy or expensive. If you prefer using technology then it is OK to carry out this activity electronically; however, I recommend going old-school and using a pen and paper if you can.

This item is going to become a personal resource called a Gratitude Diary.

At roughly the same time each day (so it becomes a habit), make a notation in your Gratitude Diary with the date of the prior day. Then in no more than ten words, write down something good about the day. There is no need to stress yourself out trying to pick the best thing that happened (the exercise isn't meant to create stress), just something that was good.

Fill in the diary every day. If you miss an entry, think back to the day(s) you have missed (you will find you can usually remember something that stands out) and make a notation.

Over a period of time, you will create a narrative of positive things happening in your life. Review your notations on a regular basis. Hopefully, you will find that the notations help you feel good about your life. Hopefully, you will also find that your sources of gratitude are diverse; that is, your sources of gratitude aren't confined to one or two aspects of your life.

Once you have done this over a year, you will have an interesting, nostalgic, and powerful source of good memories to reflect on and celebrate.

To give you an insight into how it might look, shown below are notations from my personal Gratitude Diary over two years (written on the same date—the 6th—of each month):

11/6 Crab sandwich

12/6 Two emus at dam in the Western Desert

1/6 Spanish dinner to celebrate wedding

2/6 Black cockatoos flying overhead

3/6 Repairing paddock fence damaged by floods

4/6 Writing novel, Coincidence

5/6 Walking in bush

6/6 Rainbow over property

7/6 Moving furniture for my daughter, Brianna

8/6 Chicken soup

9/6 Cutting firewood

10/6 Taking Mum and Dad to a garden nursery

11/6 *Jacaranda trees blooming in Grafton*

12/6 *Tour of Hoi An, Vietnam*

1/6 *Lunch at Hunter Vineyards restaurant for wedding anniversary*

2/6 *Feedback from participants in a workshop I delivered*

3/6 *Giving a person a headband I made out of lomandra [a native
plant used for making rope]*

4/6 *Stars*

5/6 *48mm of rain*

6/6 *Visiting cultural site with my sons, Rhys and Liam*

7/6 *Watching movie*—Best Exotic Marigold Hotel

8/6 *Sea breeze as I walked down a Brisbane street*

9/6 *New shutters for house*

10/6 *Planting vegetable garden*

By focusing on gratitude for what we have, our tendency to want
what we don't have is lessened. We live in a consumer society. The
capitalist imperative to drive demand for goods and services means
that wherever we look we are inundated with advertising telling
us to buy. The internet, social media, magazines, television, radio,
newspapers, and roadsides abound with messaging and images
telling us how much happier we will be if we purchase product Y.
Having worked in a marketing role in my life, I am aware of the focus
on creating consumer wants.

The various promotional triggers are tapping into desire,
which can easily take us to a path of greed and away from the
path of gratitude. We are being emotionally triggered, mentally
manipulated, and socially engineered to want more and more.
Will endless wanting make us happy? The answer is no. Endless
wanting will take us in the opposite direction of happiness. Endless

wanting will create a thirst that will never be quenched and will make us restless and unhappy. A far better road to contentment is to break the habit of wanting and replace it with a habit of giving. Can you imagine a world of giving rather than a world of wanting?

Exercise: What Does Giving Mean to Me?

Listed below are a number of quotes related to giving. Review each of them and, on a blank piece of paper, write down words that resonate with you.

Remember the happiest people are not those getting more, but those giving.

    —H. JACKSON BROWN, JR.

You have not lived today until you have done something for someone who can never repay you.

    —JOHN BUNYAN

We make a living by what we get. We make a life by what we give.

    —WINSTON S. CHURCHILL

There is no exercise better for the heart than reaching down and lifting people up.

    —JOHN HOLMES

For it is in giving that we receive.

    —ST. FRANCIS OF ASSISI

Always give without remembering and always receive without forgetting.

    —BRIAN TRACY

The meaning of life is to find your gift. The purpose of life is to give it away.

—PABLO PICASSO

You can give without loving, but you cannot love without giving.

—AMY CARMICHAEL

Don't judge each day by the harvest you reap, but by the seeds you plant.

—ROBERT LOUIS STEVENSON

Now write a sentence or paragraph that reflects what giving means to you. How will you convert this sentence into practice?

Think of television footage you have seen of people on city streets giving free hugs. Some people might feel uncomfortable about this, but in the majority of cases the images show myriad smiling faces and, as observers, most of us smile along with them. The joy of giving is infectious. The act of sharing goodwill and affection can grow very quickly if the seeds are planted and watered. It might be time to awaken the gardener within. Let's start a worldwide groundswell of sharing love and gratitude, and give some balance back to the planet!

There are many people involved in giving industries, working either professionally or as volunteers. They are continually giving love and goodwill. When they look back on their day, week, year, or life, they might question what they have achieved, but they have every reason to feel good about themselves. They have shared and they have cared. Without knowing it, they have been following the Lore.

Think about how your story will read when your time on this earth is almost finished. Do you want your story to be one of sharing and love? Will people describe you as giving, caring, considerate, supportive, nurturing, and loving, or will they describe you as self-centered, negative, cold, bitter, ungrateful, and angry? Look at your story right now. Are you on the right path? The opposite of love is hate, a highly destructive way of thinking and being. Some people argue that the technological advances in communications have increased the ability for some people to promote hate. In June 2020, the United Nations launched its Strategy and Plan of Action on Hate Speech in response to the alarming trends of growing xenophobia, racism and intolerance, violent misogyny, anti-Semitism, and anti-Muslim hatred around the world. So hate is something requiring our urgent attention.

Hate shares characteristics with several other negative emotions, especially anger, and builds on strong feelings of annoyance, displeasure, and hostility.

On any given day, we are surrounded by potential triggers of these emotions. Traffic lights, traffic jams, bills, mortgages, making mistakes, fear of losing our jobs, cold coffee, people letting us down, not getting enough sleep, our minds not being able to relax, slow internet speeds, being put on hold on the telephone, running late for something, having to rush, technology breakdowns—these and many other things are opportunities to be angry.

Anger is a primary emotion (along with fear, happiness, and sadness) and can be the body's first response to something happening around us. Some theorists suggest that these emotions are somewhat innate, universal, and hardwired into our brains.

Everyone feels angry sometimes. If we harness our anger in a wise way, we can use it to express how we are feeling, cope with difficult situations, and make positive changes in our lives. If, during the course of our day, we have an experience that makes us angry, the anger itself is not a problem. It is what we do with the anger that matters.

If we reflect on the anger and do something positive with the experience—take constructive action, challenge our self-talk, practice accepting and letting go of the anger, or use the situation to learn something about ourselves—then the experience doesn't impair our well-being. If we act out on the anger in a negative way, such as becoming abusive, physically assaulting someone (or ourselves), or stockpiling it, we are potentially undermining our well-being. Anger becomes a problem when it begins to negatively impact our daily life.

If we hold on to the anger, it can consume us and become an overwhelming state of mind. We might become labeled an angry ant because we seem to be always angry or on the verge of "blowing a gasket" or "losing our cool." People may start to avoid us and our relationships might suffer, which can further feed the anger bubble we have constructed.

Anger channeled the wrong way for too long can turn into hate . . . and hate is a toxic and destructive state that poisons the soul. It has caused immeasurable pain and suffering to humanity for thousands of years. It is a sad reality that at times people embrace hate rather than reject it.

Some people hate others, some people hate themselves, and in some cases, people hate both others and themselves. When we hate, we disconnect and take ourselves away from the Dreaming

Path and undermine our ability to live a good story. In doing this we are undermining our happiness and ability to maintain well-being. How can you have a good relationship with your place and all things in your place if you are disconnected by hate?

In the hundreds of Aboriginal languages that existed on this continent for tens of thousands of years, there is no word for hate and there are no stories about hate, indicating it was not a feeling that Aboriginal people encountered.

Why was there no word for hate? Have a look at the Australian landscape. Can you see any evidence of hate? If you go to Europe, you will see castles with high walls with moats around them with drawbridges. Some are even built on high cliffs. This is because in their world people fought each other and tried to take what belonged to somebody else. This created hate and animosity between peoples.

We know this didn't happen in Australia—because there wasn't one dominant language or one dominant people. Aboriginal people didn't hate—because of respect, because of love, and because of responsibility.

Hate was a concept alien to Aboriginal people for many reasons, including:

- the strength, number, and diversity of relationships;
- the respect for, and tolerance of, difference;
- commitment to the Lore; and
- the many systems that were in place for addressing anger and preventing it from escalating into hatred.

When tribal groups were traveling across Country to conduct big ceremony, there were several places along the way called "sit down" places, where people were reminded by the Elders to sit down and discuss anything they were upset about. This was done to ensure people were entering the sacred ceremony grounds with their spirits clean of any negative emotions. It was considered of utmost importance that people didn't contaminate these special areas with bad energy.

In day-to-day life, if a problem arose between two people, there were mechanisms in place to deal with the situation. Mechanism one was an expectation for the two parties to sort out any issues between themselves in a non-emotive and constructive manner. If resolution wasn't achieved, mechanism two was for Elders to support both parties in a bipartisan way until the matter was addressed.

Problems between groups were very rare. If this situation arose, Elders from each of the groups would arrange a ritualistic battle involving aggressive body posturing and actions such as the throwing of spears accompanied by verbal threats and insults. This allowed the persons involved to physically and emotionally act out their anger. When the Elders from both parties deemed it appropriate (or when blood was spilled), the battle would cease and the matter considered finished business (as was the case when conflict between individuals was resolved). Finished business meant the matter was never to be raised again. In today's world there are numerous examples of anger, hatred, and war between groups and nations. Is this a good thing for anyone? What can you or I do about this, given we are each one person in a world of more than 7.7 billion? While we may not be able to change the world, maybe we can have a positive impact on our family, our workplace, and our local community?

A starting point is understanding how to manage our anger in a healthy way. Consider these strategies:

- seeking help from a health professional
- recognizing when you are angry and reflecting on why you are angry
- taking time out when you feel yourself getting angry
- talking to someone
- practicing relaxation techniques (meditation, mindfulness, yoga)
- exercising
- balancing your anger with an appreciation of the positive things that surround you

Exercise: 10/10 Moments

Each day, if we remember to notice, there are things we can taste, see, smell, feel, hear, and experience that give us joy or delight. I call these "10/10 moments."

As you read these words, stop for a minute or two and identify three 10/10 moments that have happened to you today.

Don't stop until you have identified three (people often say, "I haven't had a 10/10 moment this month"... but once they start thinking more deeply, they usually come up with one... then the others follow relatively quickly).

Once you have done this, reflect on the two questions below:

Question 1. Did any of the 10/10 moments you identified require a large amount of money?

Question 2. Did any of the 10/10 moments you identified require a great amount of planning, organizing, and time?

You will find that, in most instances, 10/10 moments are free or inexpensive and 10/10 moments are spontaneous. If these moments are not costly and if these moments are not complex to create, why don't we have lots of them every day? The answer is we do! We just forget to look for them.

So now you know how easy it is to identify a 10/10 moment, every night, before you go to bed, contact someone verbally. It could be your partner or it could be a good friend (you can do it face-to-face or you can do it over the phone).

Explain to them the concept of 10/10 moments and ask them if they would be happy to help you carry out this exercise. If they agree, ask them to identify three 10/10 moments they had during the day. After they have shared them with you, it is your turn to share your three 10/10 moments for the day. Notice how you feel once you have done this.

When you are finished, thank them for their support and ask them if they are able to do the same task each night for fourteen nights.

After two weeks of doing this, what do you think might happen? You might find you start looking forward to sharing your 10/10s every night. You might find you start noticing 10/10s in real time. If you start noticing them in real time, you might find that each day you will start seeing more than three.

If your day becomes a day filled with 10/10 moments, how do you think you will feel at the end of each day, all things considered?

Although traditional Aboriginal people faced hardship on occasions, they had the knowledge, skills, and spiritual beliefs to accept these situations and not give in to negative mindsets. Celebrating the many good things that surrounded them helped them maintain a positive attitude toward life and reinforced the cornerstone value of humility.

Of the many values considered imperative in traditional Aboriginal life (love, respect, humility, and always sharing), from my lived experience, humility is the hardest to master. When you look at how the Western world functions, it is not hard to see why humility is such a difficult garment to wear.

A characteristic central to capitalism is the competitive market. After we battle each other at school and to get a job, we are then engaged in a system where businesses battle each other (locally and globally) to gain a competitive advantage in the marketplace in order to maintain viability or grow. Governments (the group of people with the authority to set the rules for a country or state) actively support and promote this competition, arguing that market forces ensure efficiency and keep prices down. But keeping prices down comes at a cost.

To win at school, we are encouraged to stand out. That is not being humble. To win a job in a labor market where there might be a hundred applicants for one position, we are told to sell ourselves. That is not being humble. To keep our business going, we must ensure we shine more brightly than others in our industry. That is not being humble.

There are schools, recruitment activities, and businesses that are exceptions, of course, but as an overarching system, the Western system rewards the loud and proud. The quiet achiever can often become invisible. To be humble in an environment that rewards a degree of pretension and conceit can undermine a person's ability to access important opportunities in their life and their ability to support themselves and those they love. The pressure to be seen, the pressure to stand out, the pressure to be the chosen one can result in us trying to be something that we aren't. This can incur a major personal cost. I should know. Trying to be something I wasn't nearly cost me my life.

To be humble can therefore be a big challenge as we try to carry out our many responsibilities. The question therefore arises: Is it possible to live in a humble way, pursue a career, *and* run a successful business? Bringing the two worlds, the Aboriginal and the Western, together can be done, but it requires thought, commitment, and continual review. Our Old People tell us that as we start to succeed in life, it is very easy to leave the path of humility and go down the path of inflated ego.

A long time ago, back in the Ngurrampaa, there was a bird called Gillah. He was a gray bird and he had a good friend named Garnie. Garnie was a smooth-skinned skink lizard.

Garnie was a show-off. He loved to throw his boomerang and he was really good at it. He loved to tell everybody how good he was. He would sing out, "Come over here, everybody, and watch me throw my boomerang, because I am the best boomerang thrower in the whole world." The people would say, "Be quiet, Garnie. We know you are a good boomerang thrower but we are sick of hearing it from you." His friend Gillah used to say to him, "Garnie, I will watch you because you are my good friend."

One day Garnie said, "Gillah, I will throw my boomerang at you but don't worry: I won't hit you. I will make my boomerang do three loops around your head and then it will come back to me."

Gillah said in reply, "Garnie, we have been taught not to throw things at each other. Don't throw your boomerang at me. It might hit me."

"No. I won't hit you, Gillah. I am the best in the world at boomerang throwing," Garnie replied. He threw his boomerang at Gillah. The boomerang did two circles around Gillah's head and on the third revolution it hit poor Gillah on the top of his head and sliced off the top part of his scalp.

Gillah flew away like a mad bird, shaking his head and screeching in pain. As he flew, the blood flowed from his head onto his chest and onto his wings. Since that time and to this day, Gillah is now a gray-and-pink bird from the blood that flowed from his head.

Gillah was angry and hurt by what his best friend had done and wanted payback and revenge. One day, when Garnie was walking along the side of a hill, Gillah flew down and punched Garnie in the back. Garnie fell over and rolled down the hill into all the thorns that were down in the valley. The thorns stuck in his back everywhere and he was in pain but he couldn't pull the thorns out.

He went down to the river to have a drink and saw his

*reflection in the water. He was ashamed of how ugly he looked
with the thorns sticking out of his back. He was so ashamed,
he walked off into the desert and hid under a rock, and now
he is known as the thorny devil lizard who hides because of his
ugliness.*

*From one egotistical action, thinking he was the best
boomerang thrower in the world, Garnie harmed his friend
Gillah and changed the way Gillah looked. Gillah took revenge
and now Garnie doesn't look like he did and is ashamed of how
he now looks. All this happened because of ego.*

To master humility, we need to have a strong sense of who
we are—a strong sense of self. This is not easy in a world that,
from when we are very young, inundates us with messaging re-
garding how we need to look and how we need to act in order to
be accepted, be liked, be popular, and be successful. I know this
from personal experience. As I started the process of healing
myself after my breakdown, I realized I had spent most of my
thirty-five years trying to be all things to all people at all times.
The feeling of being an outsider trying to fit in had exhausted
me to the point I wanted to end it all. Thank goodness I was
provided with an alternative pathway that enabled me to heal
and grow.

Over the past twenty-five years, I have discovered there are
many people who have a poor sense of self and are lost. They
often come up to me after I have spoken at a conference or delivered a workshop and share their relief at knowing they are not
alone. As they share their story, I can see a pattern of trauma,
vulnerability, and eroded self-confidence that has been buried for

many years. Usually, it is painted over with an ever-ready smile and outward appearance of confidence that mask pain and inner conflict which, although hidden, continue to undermine peace and contentment.

It can be hard to believe in yourself when you grow up in a society that says you must stand out but also enforces the tall poppy syndrome (a syndrome where people have a tendency to mock, discredit, or put down people who succeed). It can be hard to believe in yourself when you grow up in a society where rejection is so pervasive. It can be hard to believe in yourself if you are different from the mainstream and therefore treated differently because you don't conform.

An important stepping stone to believing in ourselves is to build our self-respect. In addition to enabling us to feel better about ourselves, building our self-respect can make a big difference to our self-esteem, how others view us, and how they treat us. The journey of respecting oneself can be a challenging one, but it is a worthy and rewarding one.

Exercise: Building Self-Respect

Listed below are a number of ways you can begin working on building your self-respect. Take as much time as you need to think about each of the items and how they relate to you. After you have done this, choose one item only and convert it into a written action that you will focus on for at least two weeks.

After two weeks have elapsed, review your progress and, if you are ready, choose another item and do the same thing. Continue working through the list (for the rest of your life if need be).

- Don't let others' opinions about you control you.
- Show respect for others.
- Identify what makes you feel good and do at least one of these things each day as a priority.
- Be in touch with your emotions and take care of your emotional needs.
- Maintain a positive attitude.
- Don't put yourself down.
- Let go of anger at those who have hurt you.
- Know yourself, accept who you are, and be true to that person.
- Believe you are worthy of respect.
- Stop trying to keep up with everyone.
- Don't let anybody force you to be or do anything you don't want to be or do simply to gain their approval.
- Be friendly.
- Don't compare yourself to others, try to fit in, or try to be "normal."
- Show you care.
- Cast aside envy.
- Don't do things that are against your values, morals, or ethics.
- Connect with positive people.
- Learn to say no.
- Work on building your confidence.
- Trust your choices.
- Never stop learning.
- Be truthful.
- Remind yourself that whatever you do today is enough.
- Learn to deal with criticism.
- Connect with something spiritual.

- Make good decisions.
- Don't let the past dictate your present.
- Don't let others get to you.
- Accept your responsibilities.
- Say sorry.
- Don't rely on others to feel good about yourself.
- Learn to accept compliments.
- Look in the mirror each day and say out loud three things you love about yourself.
- Admit when you are wrong.
- Focus on your positive traits.
- Stay humble.
- Forgive yourself.

As you build your self-respect, you build your ability for self-love. It can be hard to be self-loving when often self-loving can be labeled as selfish. It is important to acknowledge to yourself that being self-loving is not the same as being selfish. In Aboriginal culture, loving yourself is respecting that you are conceived in love, born in love, and living in love. Loving yourself is an important element of loving your place and all things in your place. By loving who we are and believing in ourselves, we are in a far better position to walk our footsteps and live a good story. The process of falling in love can be a powerful experience.

Falling in love with yourself is therefore something to welcome. It starts with reflecting on how you think—reflecting on the self-talk generated inside your head.

The human brain is a magnificent ally. With it we reflect,

learn, solve problems, stay alive, feel joy, give love, and receive love. It can also be a powerful and persuasive enemy if we allow it to flood our being with negative self-talk. When we do this, we fuel self-doubt that can undermine our confidence and chain us to damaging self-labels, such as "I am an imposter," "I am unlovable," "I am stupid," or "I need to be a success." I have placed these labels on myself several times.

When we start believing these labels, we can find ourselves adopting submissive behaviors in a situation or relationship where we are unconsciously saying, "Your needs count and mine don't." In this kind of situation, we are undermining our self-worth. We are not embracing love for ourselves and not valuing our essence. We are not walking our own footsteps.

Alternatively, when we start believing these labels, we can find ourselves adopting aggressive behaviors in a situation or relationship where we are unconsciously saying, "My needs count and yours don't." This kind of interaction is also highly counterproductive. We might get our way in the short term, but ultimately people will disconnect from us and our relationships will wither and die.

When we see these labels for what they are (untrue responses to things that have happened in our life), we can adopt a far more productive headspace if in a situation or relationship we say, "Your needs count and so do mine." With this kind of mindset, we are respecting the other person and also respecting ourselves. It is a win-win attitude.

As you build your self-respect and self-love and begin to connect to the real you, be warned: ego will not want to end its former, unhealthy relationship with you.

That ego is very tricky. He is also really stubborn. He won't want to leave you, so he will disguise himself so you might not see him. You might be planning to do something good for others and your ego will say to you, "You are doing the right thing. So go ahead and do it." But deep down inside you know you are doing it so you can be noticed. Ego has won.

But you might be planning to do something good for others and you're not really worried if anybody knows about what you have done. In this case, you have done it for the right reasons and ego has not had any part to play. So when you are doing something, ask yourself, am I doing this because it is the right thing to do, or am I doing it because I want to be noticed?

How often do we see egotistical and arrogant behavior from others? When we see this behavior, how does it make us feel? When a person is behaving in an egotistical or arrogant way, they are sending the message "I am more important than you." This contradicts the Lore, which tells us we are all equally important. It is critical we don't buy in to this kind of behavior by saying to ourselves something like "They are more important than me, so I had better do what they say" or "They are obviously smarter than me, so I had better not disagree." This kind of self-talk can undermine our self-belief and compromise our feelings of self-worth.

Unpacking what we are thinking where necessary and challenging our negative self-talk mitigates the risk we'll create harmful mind chatter that can lead us down the path of "awfulizing." Rather than looking at a given incident objectively and accepting it for what it is, "awfulizers" add to their angst by telling themselves how "awful" the situation is. This kind of thinking significantly adds to their disquiet and takes them further away from peace, serenity, and calm.

By challenging our negative thought patterns and looking at situations more objectively, we are better able to:

- take ownership of our life,
- choose the actions we want to carry out in a given situation,
- channel our energy into the right things, and
- reduce the tension we may feel at a moment in time.

Not that tension is always a bad thing. Many people see tension and challenge in their lives as things to be avoided. This can be a mistake. Challenge and tension can be productive forces. They can be a catalyst for personal change.

If we feel tension, it may be a message that there is something wrong in our life. By reflecting on why we are feeling tense, we might identify something we need to change. This might challenge us, but rather than shy away from the challenge, it might be useful to assess whether the change is something worthwhile.

Challenges are opportunities to learn. They can motivate us to take stock of our life, to reflect on, identify, and execute changes that will benefit us. By challenging habitually negative thoughts, for example, we can reshape our internal storylines and give ourselves new ways of viewing the world and how we behave in it. Looking back at my life, some of my greatest challenges have given me my greatest opportunities for personal growth and life satisfaction.

Changing a lifetime of habit in the way we label ourselves and behave in specific situations is not easy. Physiologically, the brain can take years to rewire neural pathways to the new way of thinking, so, as you embark on this journey, it is important to be patient.

We live in a fast-paced society that seems to test our patience rather than nurture it. But a masterpiece is rarely created in a day, and *you* are a masterpiece—a work in progress. Creating the best possible you will take time. It will also involve trial and error. Be patient and welcome the mistakes you will inevitably make on your road to improved well-being. Acknowledge them as your friend as they will give you opportunities to learn and practice what you have learned.

The more you achieve, the more you will make mistakes. The more you make mistakes, the more you will reflect. The more you reflect, the more you will learn. The more you learn, the more you will grow. The more you grow, the more you will share. The more you share, the more you will connect. The more you connect, the more you will achieve . . . and so the cycle goes on.

If you find yourself struggling at times to embrace love, gratitude, and humility, don't give up or condemn yourself. Instead, investigate what is happening, what you can learn from what is happening, and what you need to do differently.

You are loved by the Mother, the Father, and the Spirit Ancestors. They want you to live a good story. By living your life with love, gratitude, and humility, you are in a better position to do just that.

Message 6

We are conceived in love, born into love, and surrounded by love. The love of the Mother, the Father, and the Spirit Ancestors is always there for us.

Message 7

Carry out loving deeds for others and yourself as often as you can.

Message 8

Give thanks every day for the abundance of good things that surround you.

Message 9

Be humble in all you do.

Chapter 4

Learning and Truth

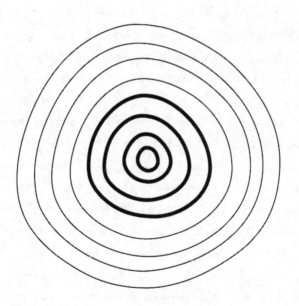

Way back in the Ngurrampaa, there was a Grandfather Eagle who lived in a cave on the top of a small rocky hill surrounded by the most beautiful trees and plants.

Grandfather Eagle was an Elder in his community who had great love for his people. He particularly loved his two nephews, Magpie and Crow, who often stayed with him.

Way back in the Ngurrampaa, Magpie and Crow were both white birds. They were so white they almost glowed in the dark. Magpie and Crow loved how they looked.

They also loved spending time with Grandfather Eagle, because at the bottom of the small rocky hill where he lived was a creek full of mussels, oysters, crayfish, and other food. When Magpie and Crow weren't eating food from the creek, they would spend all day eating lots of vegetables and fruit from the bush next to the creek.

Whenever they went to Grandfather Eagle's camp, they would barely say hello before quickly making their way down to the creek to play. This used to frustrate Grandfather Eagle a great deal, as he knew the boys were growing into young men and he had a responsibility to teach them the Lore so they could fulfill their responsibilities when the time came.

"Come here, my nephews," he would say in the gentlest of voices. "I need to take you on Country and show you things so you can learn."

"Yes, Grandfather," they would reply. "We know we need to listen to you so we can learn, but not today. It is a good day to go down to the creek and we must go." And Magpie and Crow would leave without waiting for Grandfather Eagle's response.

This used to hurt Grandfather Eagle a great deal and also worry him. "I have an obligation to share knowledge with these boys," he would say to himself as he perched on his small rocky hill that looked over the most beautiful trees and plants. "But they will not listen to me. I must do something about this. If I don't, I will be failing them and I will not be fulfilling my responsibilities. I know what I will do. I will call a meeting with the other animals and share my worry with them. Between us we will come up with a solution."

So old Grandfather Eagle called a meeting of the animals and, because he was such a well-respected and loved Elder, they all came. There were all sorts of animals, including pelicans, owls, possums, snakes, lizards, kangaroos, koalas, goannas, echidnas, emus, and bandicoots at the gathering. Grandfather Eagle told them of his worry and they all agreed that something needed to be done. They had been concerned about Magpie and Crow as well.

"Grandfather, it is not just your obligation to ensure these boys have the knowledge to become good young men," Owl said. "We all share that obligation. We will all help you."

The animals sat around for hours and hours sharing ideas until eventually they all agreed on what needed to be done. After the meeting had finished, all the animals said goodbye to Grandfather Eagle and told him they loved him. That evening, Grandfather Eagle watched the most beautiful of sunsets and gave thanks for the Country he lived on and the community he lived with.

Finally the day came to carry out the plan they had agreed on. It was an hour or so before sunset and all the animals started to arrive at Grandfather Eagle's camp. Each animal brought with them some firewood and some food because they knew it wasn't right to take food and wood from Grandfather Eagle's place and leave him with nothing.

As they arrived, Grandfather Eagle hugged each of them and then asked each animal to put the firewood at the front of the cave and the food at the back of the cave. His nephews were, as always, playing in the creek below and so had no idea the animals were gathering at Grandfather Eagle's camp.

Eventually all the animals had arrived for the corroboree. The emus started dancing around the fire and had all the animals laughing as they stomped and did a "shake-a-leg." Other animals followed and before long the sound of clapsticks, singing, and laughter filled the valley where Magpie and Crow were playing. Magpie was the first to notice. "Hey. What's that noise?" he said as he lifted his head and looked toward the top of the hill.

Berries fell out of his full mouth as he spoke. He and Crow had been eating all day.

"Sounds like a corroboree," Crow replied. "We should head up. Bet there's lots of tucker."

They flew to the top of the hill as fast as they could. When they reached Grandfather Eagle's cave, they saw the animals gathered around the dancing circle outside the cave, but they were far more interested in the smell of food coming from inside the cave.

They hurried past the animals without saying hello to anyone and without paying respects to their Elders. Grandfather Eagle shook his head with sadness as he watched them.

Within minutes, Magpie's and Crow's faces were buried in the food the animals had placed at the back of the cave. They were so busy eating, they didn't notice that the animals had stopped dancing and were now standing in front of the stack of wood at the cave's entrance.

Grandfather Eagle nodded to Kangaroo, who hopped over from a corroboree fire with a firestick and set the stack of wood alight. In no time, the entire stack was ablaze, filling the cave with smoke, but Magpie and Crow didn't notice.

More time passed and the smoke became thicker. Eventually Magpie lifted his beak from a bowl of plums and sniffed loudly. "Hey . . . Crow . . . I can smell smoke."

Crow ignored him. He was too busy eating.

Magpie turned around and saw the fire and became scared. "Crow," he said. "The cave's on fire. I'm getting out of here." Magpie flew out of the cave but the flames were everywhere. As he landed outside the cave, many of his feathers were alight. Thankfully the animals were waiting outside and they were able to put the flames out quickly.

"Gee, this tucker is really good, ay?" Crow said, lifting his head and then noticing that Magpie wasn't there. He saw how thick the smoke had become and turned around to see the bright orange of the fire covering the entire entrance to the cave. Crow panicked and immediately flew through the flames. The flames were so fierce that all his feathers caught alight, but thankfully the animals were waiting outside and they were able to put the flames out quickly.

After things had calmed down and the animals were able to reassure Magpie and Crow that they weren't badly hurt, Magpie and Crow looked at each other.

"Look at you, Magpie." Crow laughed. "You are no longer white . . . you are Black and white."

"Well, you think that's funny," Magpie replied with a growl. "You should see yourself. You have no white at all. You are entirely Black."

Both Magpie and Crow started to cry loudly as they walked over to Grandfather Eagle.

"Grandfather," they said, sobbing. "We know you are wise and talk to the sky father. Can you ask him to come down? We want our beautiful white feathers back."

Biamii, the sky father, had been watching all that had happened and appeared before Grandfather Eagle could reply. "Listen here," Biamii said in the sternest of voices, which made Magpie and Crow start crying again.

"Listen here, you boys. Your grandfather has tried to get you to travel Country with him many times so he can fulfill his obligations and teach you the Lore. He does this because he loves you, not because he wants to annoy you. But every time he has tried, you have ignored him. So you have not learned to be respectful, and you have not learned to be humble."

Magpie's and Crow's crying became louder as Biamii continued. "You have not learned to love all things. You are greedy boys." Magpie's and Crow's crying was now so loud the animals had to cover their ears. "From this day on, Magpie, you will be a black-and-white bird, to remind you and everybody around you of the need to listen to your Elders so you can learn the Lore. And Crow, you will forever be a black bird, to remind you and everybody around you of the need to listen to your Elders so you can learn the Lore."

And to this day, sometimes if you look up into the sky, you might see an eagle being followed by a magpie and a crow. And if you were able to hear them speaking, you would hear Magpie and Crow still telling Grandfather Eagle how sorry they are for not respecting him and not learning about the Lore.

The Lore tells us we must care for our place and all things in our place and provides us with the knowledge of how to do this. The way we gain knowledge is through the learning process, which involves acquiring information and combining it with what we experience to transform how we view the world.

In traditional Aboriginal Australia, learning was a lifelong process integrated into all aspects of daily life to ensure all community members were able to fulfill their individual and community responsibilities.

In our modern world, the school system is seen as a compulsory and critical part of our growth from young child to young adult. Although the importance of learning is acknowledged as the foundation for future well-being, for many, the school experience is an unpleasant and damaging one.

A respect for learning, a love of learning, and the ability to be a self-directed lifelong learner are essentials if we are to live a good story. If our experience of learning in our younger years is a negative one, we are less likely to engage in the accrual of knowledge that is essential for us to navigate adult life, fulfill our responsibilities, achieve our goals, and find a place of contentment. Listing the various types of learning methodology demonstrates how complex the learning process can be. There is active learning, play, nonassociative learning, enculturation, episodic learning, multimedia learning, rote learning, meaningful learning, evidence-based learning, formal learning, informal learning, tangential learning, dialogue learning, and incidental learning practices for the teacher to navigate, contemplate, and possibly use in the teaching and learning process. Is it any wonder that this can be such a difficult experience for both the teacher and the young person?

The Aboriginal learning system, although sophisticated in terms of the use of integrated learning methodologies and theory, is built on a simple premise: the importance of looking and listening.

The more we look and listen, the more we learn. The Old People would say things like, "Now, if you come to me knowing everything, I can teach you nothing, but if you come to me knowing nothing, I can teach you everything." You have to come with humility. You have to come ready to listen. You have to come ready to look. Otherwise you won't learn anything.

From the day we are born, we are programmed to look and listen. This is how we grow our awareness and build our knowledge base. It is an innate way of being for us as children.

In traditional Aboriginal life, looking, listening, and learning provided a continuous educational experience that complemented learning activities such as being shown how to do a specific task, visiting a site, or being given a story while sitting around the fire at night.

An important component of the learning process was the use of silence. Aboriginal people to this day are very comfortable with silence. It is something that can be unnerving to people who are used to a world where constant sound invades their ears, visual imagery saturates their eyes, and information overload inundates their brain. This world of hyperstimulation is somewhat different from the traditional Aboriginal world, where we relax softly into the subtle sounds of nature and allow the quiet to open our eyes and ears to an infinite classroom of learning that surrounds us.

The way we learn about people's stories is by looking and listening. Sitting down with one another, listening to one another, looking at what the Old People are showing us, looking at what the land is showing us, what the animals are showing us, listening to the land, watching the land: we grow by looking and listening.

To train our eyes and ears to actively watch and hear, the Old People tell us how important it is to walk Country in a connected way, taking in all that is around us.

Walking Country is a practice that enables us to:

- remember the importance of nature;
- connect with nature;
- connect with family;

- connect with spirit;
- connect with ourselves;
- reflect on our life journey;
- be still;
- be mindful;
- feel loved; and
- look, listen, and learn.

Listening to Country can change our lives. Listening to others can change our lives. Listening to others can change their lives. So listening is a good skill to work on.

If you are with a person and they are talking to you, although it is important to observe their body language and facial movements, be sure to listen with all that you have. Listen to the words, listen to the tone of voice, and listen to the story that is being told.

It is also important to listen to yourself. To do this, you need quiet to surround you and you need quiet within you. In this place of quiet, it is important to listen deeply to your sacred self, your intuitive self, your true self.

Listening can give us amazing insights into what is happening around us. No matter where you live, listening to the sounds of life can be a wonderful thing to do.

Hear the sound of the breeze in the trees as the leaves rustle in a beautiful collective dance. What can you learn from this sound? To dance with spirit.

Hear the welcome sound of rain after a drought. What can you learn from this sound? To always remember how water gives life to all things.

Listen to the sound of a baby crying down the street. What can you learn from this sound? To take the time to say hello to new parents and be there for them should they need a break.

Notice the sound of your partner telling you about their day. What can you learn from this sound? To be thankful for having someone who trusts you enough to share their day and their life with you.

A car has just screamed past. The motor is revving loudly. What can you learn from this sound? To not make assumptions. The car might be driven by someone who is irresponsible, or the driver might be trying to get someone to the hospital in a life-and-death situation.

There are numerous opportunities to practice listening—podcasts, at work, in class, in a social setting, at home, out walking, when you are meditating, or when someone is sharing their soul one-on-one with you. When we commit to listening, it is important that we commit our entire attention. Stop texting or scrolling on your phone, turn the phone off, stop thinking about other things, empty the mind, and really focus on what you are hearing. If it is with another person, respect them enough to stop what you are doing, create the space to connect, let everything else slip into the background, and be there for them. Ten minutes of "being there" could be more important than you ever imagined. You can use the process outlined above when you look around you. When you look at things, as long as it is appropriate to do so, look at them with depth and great interest. Observe as if you were looking at this object or person for the first time. Notice color, texture, shape, movement. Allow yourself to be lost in the wonder of sight. As you do, you will be taken into another world of learning.

Looking and listening can involve far more than using your eyes and ears. Look and listen with your body . . . look and listen with your spirit . . . look and listen with your intuition.

We look and listen in order to gain knowledge so we can better connect with what is around us. If we connect with what is around us, we learn. If we learn, we grow. If we grow, we find meaning. If we find meaning, we have purpose. If we have purpose, we are better able to fulfill our potential. If we fulfill our potential, we find contentment. Looking, listening, and learning are therefore critical elements to achieving contentment and well-being.

In traditional Aboriginal society there was compulsory schooling, but it was very different from the modern-day school. Instead of students being channeled into a classroom, an Aboriginal student's classroom was the bush . . . an ever-expanding, interactive, ever-changing learning space where the classroom could be around a fire, in a clearing, under a tree, at the beach, on a rock platform, on a riverbed . . . anywhere that would reinforce the lesson being given.

Knowledge was transferred in a variety of ways, including storytelling, song, dance, art, and walking Country. The learning process involved all members of the community (as learners and educators) and embodied a number of key characteristics considered good practice today.

The traditional learning model:

- provided a nurturing environment;
- had 100 percent student participation;
- was lifelong and continuous;
- used blended and flexible delivery modes;
- incorporated technical, soft, and life skills;

- combined practical and theoretical elements;
- was customized and individualized to student need;
- involved stepped competency development, starting at a beginner level and increasing skill level over time;
- was quality assessed; and
- aimed to provide the student with everything they needed for a successful transition into adult life and beyond.

How many of these characteristics do you think are embedded in current educational delivery systems? How many of these characteristics were embedded in your learning experience? What difference do you think it would make locally, nationally, and globally if these characteristics were integrated into all learning? For many of us, if we look back at our school experience, we might wish we had done things differently, but we might also wish the system had been different. Compared to the Aboriginal learning system, the Western learning system falls short in a number of ways.

If an athlete isn't able to prepare properly for competition, how can they perform at their best? If a builder hasn't been trained in all elements of construction, would you contract them to build your house? If a child hasn't been given the right preparation for adult life, how smooth or effective will their transition be?

You can succeed despite not being provided with the right learning early in your life, of course, but it is much better to get it right in the first instance.

The Aboriginal learning system was taught every day by family. The learning process occurred pretty well twenty-four hours a day, seven days a week.

*The Aboriginal learning system was all about what you
needed for a good life, not what you wanted. When you
learned how to collect fruit from a tree, it wasn't about just
you, but who you had to share it with. When you learned how
to hunt and kill a kangaroo, it was about you and who you
shared it with. So attached to all learning was obligation and
responsibility.*

*But before you could collect fruit or kill a kangaroo you had
to learn the story of the kangaroo or the fruit and learn the
story of its ancestral path and how you have responsibilities
to them. Part of this was knowing the story, knowing the
dance and knowing the song of this ancestor before you could
partake.*

Because the Aboriginal learning system is holistic in nature, all learning is infused with spirituality. It honors the past by teaching students about the Lore and the importance of the Spirit Ancestors, connects to the present by teaching students how to harvest what is around them in the here and now, and provides for the future by preparing the student for adult life.

Early schooling in the Western system aims to support the child to build a sense of self, as was the case in traditional times. The child's development—physical, social, emotional, and cognitive—is nurtured in numerous creative ways.

As the child moves through the primary years and into the secondary years, the amount of effort required to continue building the student's physical, social, emotional, and cognitive capability can become burdensome on a learning system with finite resources. This is where the Western system starts to diverge from the Aboriginal system in terms of purpose and focus. The school system is expected to prepare students for the workforce, leading to the prioritization of technical skills, such as literacy and numeracy, mathematics, history, geography, and science, at the expense of whole-of-life skills.

Some students flourish in this learning environment, but those who don't fit in to the relatively rigid learning framework can find themselves experiencing a negative educational experience, being left behind in the assessment process, and starting to label themselves as dumb. For these students, the biggest tragedy of all is they may miss out on the opportunity to build a love of learning. A student who is given the love of learning by those around them has a lifetime asset that will enable them to look, listen, and learn in a variety of situations and contexts for the rest of their life. It is one of life's greatest gifts.

If a student disengages from the education system, their ability to successfully compete in the job market, believe in themselves, believe in their future, and establish a platform for well-being is severely impaired. Students who are successful in the education system may have the skills to get a job and generate money, which is obviously important, but do they have the skills to build contentment and fulfillment?

Financial success is not a guaranteed pathway to well-being. To achieve true prosperity, an individual must service their own emotional, physical, spiritual, and mental needs as well as financial ones. Failure to do this creates imbalance and places the person at significant risk.

The Aboriginal learning system created a pathway to contentment through the provision of technical, scientific, social, cognitive, language, physical, emotional, artistic, and spiritual skill sets that are just as important today as they have been over tens of thousands of years. By integrating mind, body, and spirit aspects into all learning activities, students are in a far better place to care for themselves, care for Country, care for others, and achieve a life of prosperity.

> Our traditional diet was 100 percent natural. It involved gathering raw plants, and the majority of our food was eaten raw. To gather food meant lots of walking and therefore exercise for the body. Diet varied according to seasons and provided great diversity.
>
> We only ever took what we needed and left the rest there for somebody else who might come along behind us. As an old man once said to me, "Never eat to be full. You should always leave a little hunger in your belly."
>
> When you leave a little hunger in your belly, you are reminded of your connection with Country and how Country provides us with all you need. You are reminded to give thanks for all that you have.

Integrating aspects of the traditional Aboriginal learning model (teaching approach, learning purpose, learning content, learning environment, and community involvement) into the Western school system would benefit not only young people. Society as a whole would benefit as well.

A young person who had built a strong sense of self in younger years would better weather the journey through adolescence to young adulthood, which can be so difficult; they would have higher self-esteem and more easily resist the pressure to fit in with peers at any cost. After learning how to build rich and enduring relationships, the young person would have a network of support for the good times and tough times ahead.

For the rest of us, there would be more jobs, increased teacher satisfaction, improved staff morale, increased community involvement, increased community connectedness, and less pressure on taxpayer-funded programs to try to address the downstream problems caused by learner disengagement.

Bringing the two worlds together is not the sole responsibility of schools. The learning system needs to be a collaboration that includes extended family and community, as has been the case in Australia for the past 60,000 years. The responsibility of changing the system belongs to us all.

If you could go back in time and visit your fourteen-year-old self at school, what advice would you give in terms of education and life? If you were made the minister for education, what changes would you make to the school system so that current fourteen-year-old students can benefit from your advice?

We can't change our past learning experiences, but we can address shortfalls from the past and build our capability for the future by assessing the opportunities formal and informal learning provide us.

Formal learning involves instruction and usually leads to a qualification. Informal learning is about what we learn through everyday experiences. Given we can do this in so many ways— such as through reading, using a computer, watching television, listening to the radio, attending public lectures, volunteering, being with family and friends, mentoring, spending time with Elders, and walking Country—informal learning is a daily opportunity too good to miss.

In my life, I have benefited from both types of learning. Formal learning has given me credibility and mobility in terms of my career while informal learning has supported my career and also enabled me to build on my passions in diverse areas, including music and healing.

Although my formal studies have been important in my life, informal learning, particularly through spending time with Elders and walking Country, has had the biggest impact on my life by far. Many people think that formal education is more important, but it depends on what you need. Just because learning is informal doesn't mean it isn't powerful. My cultural learning has been both profound and life-changing.

We are all learners and we can't live a good story without ongoing learning. If you doubt your ability to learn, start with small steps in an area you are passionate about. You might be pleasantly surprised by where the learning path takes you.

The time is right, right now, for you to consider your life journey, the role of learning in your journey, and to embrace learning in all its shapes and forms. If there are readily identifiable things you know you need to learn, now is the time to develop a plan of action and make it happen.

Our Old People teach us that the more people are involved in our learning, the richer our learning will be. It is the same when planning our learning. It is important to explore formal, nonformal, and informal opportunities for learning when considering how to best build your toolbox of knowledge.

Exercise: Whole-of-Life Learning Plan

A Learning Plan is a document that you can use to plan your learning (formal, nonformal, and informal) over an extended period of time.

Outlined below are a number of learning areas. Review them and identify three areas you would like to work on over the next year.

Learning Areas
- Physical
- Relationships
- Spiritual
- Work
- Mind
- Passion/hobbies
- Other

For each of the three learning areas you have prioritized:
- Identify what success looks like for you in that learning area (you can use pictures or words).
- Convert the pictures/words of success into a learning goal.
- Write down why the learning goal is important to you.
- Research the different learning activities you can undertake to achieve your goal (formal, nonformal, and informal).
- Select the learning activity or activities you need to undertake.
- Close your eyes and imagine how you will feel when you achieve the goal.
- Write down words to capture how you felt.

Write up a table with these headings:
- Learning area
- Goal

- Activities
- Timeline
- How I will feel when goal is achieved

This table is your Learning Plan.

Review the Learning Plan every three months. If you are on track, congratulate yourself with a special celebration. If you aren't on track, reflect on why and, if appropriate, what needs to be done to address the situation.

If you are having problems doing this on your own, identify someone who can help you.

Your Learning Plan captures an extremely personal journey. It is just as unique as you are. What you would like to learn, how you learn, the value of what you learn, and how you feel about it all come from you.

There is, and will only ever be, one you. You should never compare your learning, your knowledge, and your abilities with other people's. Comparing yourself with other people will just set you up to potentially feel like a failure.

You are just as special as anyone else, with a special road before you. So why try to compare yourself, your journey, and your learning with others? You have nothing to prove. But you do have a responsibility to be the best you that you can be. You do have a responsibility to live the best story possible. Learning is a critical catalyst for this.

In terms of how you learn, it is important for you to sample a variety of learning styles to help identify what works for you.

Some people learn better in a group environment (classroom, workshops), some learn better one-on-one (coaching, mentoring), and some prefer to learn on their own (e-learning, distance learning).

Some people are visual learners (seeing), some aural (listening), and some experiential (doing). Some like formal assignments, exams, and feedback, and some prefer to just look and reflect. Some people like to receive formal qualifications and certificates, while others aren't overly concerned about them.

In the modern world, formal qualifications are sometimes essential if you have a specific job or career in mind, but your learning shouldn't stop there. Without the assortment of knowledge you gain informally in your life, your skill base will be inadequate and you will not grow as you should. As with all things in life, diversity is important, as is balance. At the end of the day, however, what you have learned is of no use if you don't use it and if you don't share it.

The minute I stop learning is the minute I give up on life. The more I learn, the more I am able to fulfill my responsibilities.

Our Old People also teach us to be patient in our learning. Look at the land when it rains. Slow, steady, patient rain is absorbed into the land and life flourishes. Heavy, rushing rain runs over the land and out to sea, causing erosion and floods—the land becomes sick and life withers. Our learning is the same. If we take our time, knowledge is absorbed and we will flourish. If we rush, the knowledge will not sink in and we can start to think we are failing. Anxiety can arise, our confidence then slips, and we might think about giving up. If this happens, our ability to live the story we choose is at risk.

Being patient can be difficult if you believe you aren't progressing quickly enough. If this happens, focus on the distance you have traveled rather than how far there is to go. Many years ago I decided to teach myself to play the guitar. After many months, I became disillusioned and told myself I wasn't making any progress at all. A friend told me to switch the guitar around and play the chords with my other hand. When I tried to play with my "wrong" hand, it was obvious how much better I was with my "right" hand, and I realized that I had come a lot further than I had given myself credit for.

As you learn new things, you might find your understanding of long-held views on a variety of matters changes. You might also identify the need to unlearn beliefs, attitudes, and opinions you have held on to for many years. Changing old habits can be a challenge, but it is a challenge that your learning prepares you for. Getting rid of things that are holding you back will help you achieve your goals and live a good story.

Quite often, when the flame of learning has been ignited, people realize just how much they don't know about the world. This can prompt a newfound appetite for learning. If you feed this appetite with learning that balances mind, body, and spirit in a way that connects to the Ngurrampaa, you will be following the Dreaming Path and become a priceless resource for yourself, for your family, for those around you, for society, and for the earth.

As you grow as a learner and begin to share knowledge, you become a source of learning for others. This is a tremendous privilege as well as a great responsibility. It is therefore most important that the knowledge you pass on is true.

An old man once said to me, "If you don't know where you come from, you will never know where you are going." You can't just exist from today. Everything you have in your head, all the things you have in your heart or your mind, where does it come from?

It doesn't come from the future, because the future hasn't happened. It doesn't come from the present moment either. All the things you value, that you respect, that you know, come from the past. Some of the knowledge in your head comes from Socrates. Some of it comes from Einstein. Great scholars have learned things and shared that knowledge and now you have got it.

Some of this knowledge you have comes from your mum and dad, from your grandparents, from television, from the pub, or from just general conversations you had with somebody. But it all comes from the past.

How do we know if this knowledge is true? How do we know whether what we value or believe to be true is actually true? Great scholars become great scholars because they challenge what they have been taught. When they challenge, when they question, they then discover something new. Imagine if they kept this discovery to themselves? It would be a pointless thought, a pointless discovery. Knowledge is nothing if we don't share it.

It is a good thing to challenge what we are told or read and ask ourselves, "Is this truth?" Because if it is not true, we are being caught up in a lie.

The need for truth is embedded in the Lore and was a cornerstone of traditional life. There are many traditional stories that teach us the importance of telling the truth, including the thikar-billa story in Chapter 3. In contemporary society, a high value seems to be placed on truth. We are told from a young age that we shouldn't lie, yet research indicates that most adults do. We lie to cover up mistakes, for personal benefit, to be accepted, to help others, to hurt others, to avoid difficult situations, and for many other reasons. On any given day, it is likely we are going to hear lies and possibly tell them.

We therefore need to be vigilant when receiving and sharing information. This need has been heightened in recent years due in part to advancements in technology that make it relatively easy for people to spread misinformation.

We often read about scams and schemes that are trying to catch us out, but a less-thought-about problem is gossip. To gossip is to share conversations and comments about other people's private lives that are often unkind and sometimes untrue. It's a practice in which any one of us can easily become ensnared, but the act is detrimental spiritually, mentally, and emotionally to us all. When we are involved in gossip, no one wins. If and when you get trapped in a thread of gossip, ask yourself, "Do I need to hear this? Would I like it if someone was talking about me in this way? Do I want to be part of this?"

Asking ourselves if something we are being told is true is a good thing to do. It doesn't mean we have become paranoid or cynical about people. It just means that we have an awareness of the real world and how there are those who will abuse our goodwill and kindness if we aren't prudent. Although knowing when we are being told a lie is important, it can be a hard thing to identify, especially if you are by nature a very trusting person.

In trying to determine if we are being told the truth, it is important to understand that we are especially prone to accepting lies that affirm our own worldviews and ignoring information that challenges us. In addition to being careful when we hear something we like, it is also important for us to be open in our attitude when hearing something we don't like. Shutting out alternative opinions and information can prevent us from finding the truth. It can also stop us from learning and growing.

It is an unfortunate reality that the more learning we access, the greater the likelihood we are going to be provided with some inaccurate information. This is a problem for us, for our communities, for our nation, and for the world. Trying to create a home, workplace, community, nation, and world that speaks the truth will build trust and build relationships that enhance unity, goodwill, and collective well-being. It will also reflect the teachings within the Lore. This brave new world of truth-telling begins with you.

In addition to the benefits highlighted above, truth-telling also makes it easier for us to make decisions. When we make decisions, we often rely on accurate information from a variety of sources. Making a decision based on inaccurate or deliberately misleading information could mean we lose our house, lose our life savings, see a relationship suffer, feel violated, or lose our health. Living in a world where we don't know whether we are being told the truth is therefore a big problem for us individually and collectively.

Honesty was an important norm in traditional Aboriginal society and it's still something we value in the contemporary world.

It is up to each of us to demand truth from leaders, companies, the media, and people we interact with. It is also up to each of us to expose those who misinform or promulgate lies. In expecting those around us to be truthful, we also need to ensure we are doing the same thing. This includes being true to ourselves and embracing our own unique story.

When you are sitting down in a group, can you say good things about a person not there but who everybody knows? Or do you feel you have to put that person down to make yourself feel good? When you have the need to put someone else down to make yourself feel good, it means you haven't connected with your power, your inner self, your soul, your source of happiness. Your power is deep inside you. You need to find it, listen to it and act in accordance with what it tells you. This is listening to your truth.

To achieve a life of contentment, we need to live our truth. To live our truth, we need to know ourselves. To know ourselves requires us to be honest with ourselves. To do this we need to find an inner place of quiet and connect with our wise self, our intuitive self, our ancient self . . . and we need to listen.

From birth to the grave we have a multitude of entities, including family, friends, peer groups, teachers, media, religious figures, and politicians, telling us what a successful life looks like. This can become a cloud of noise that surrounds our mind and spirit, making it almost impossible to interrogate our personal truth, to identify our purpose and answer the questions, "Who am I and why do I exist?"

Exercise: Footprints in the Sand

The exercise below will help you reflect on your life so far as
to whether you are living your truth. It might help if you record
the words so you can listen to them with your eyes closed. An
alternative is to have someone read the script to you.

*Imagine you are walking barefoot along a beach. It is a beautiful
beach. On your left is an endless painting of shimmering turquoise
ocean. On your right is a mosaic of lush green rain forest. Ahead is a
golden path for you to explore. There are no people here. There is not
even a single footprint in the sand.*

*The sand is like fine powder and there is a gentle swoosh as small
waves create a melodic pulse of bliss that washes through you. The
waves are reaching out to you, wanting to connect with you, wanting
to cleanse and heal your tired soul. The sun is beaming down,
showering your skin with warmth that soaks deep into your spirit.
The sky is the most beautiful of blues. Looking at it, you think you
have never seen this color before. It is perfect. You feel like you are
looking at infinity.*

*As you observe the vastness, you feel a deep, resonating love
bathe you and you are told how important you are.*

*You slowly look around you at the beach, the water, the forest, and
the sky as you breathe in many fragrances you hadn't noticed before.
The subtlest of breezes caresses your arms, face, back, chest, and
legs. It feels so good to be alive.*

*As you walk, you feel the strain of the past few months falling
off you. The pressures of work are gone, as are the worries about
paying the bills, raising a family, eating healthy food, getting to the
gym, and trying to be a better person.*

As the present-day worries disappear, they are replaced by memories of disappointments of the past but, much to your surprise, these quickly disappear as well. They drop away with so much ease that you wonder why you hadn't done this earlier . . . and then you let that thought go as well and totally focus on the feel of the sand under your feet.

Out of nowhere, your mind starts to think about the future. A part of you says the future is going to be great, but a surprisingly loud other inner voice says this is not true. The voice is very persuasive. It tells you that you must be alert to the dangers that might befall you if you want your future to be assured.

As the warnings continue with their relentless pessimism, you find your mind floating off into the serenity that surrounds you. The inner voice's messages of doom just don't seem to be that compelling anymore.

You walk, and you walk, and you walk. The sand is warm but every now and then you step on a cooler portion of sand that sends tingles up through your feet, your neck, and into your head. The sand feels amazing. It feels so good to be just lost in the present moment. For much of your life you have wondered where you fit in, but right now, you know you are part of this place and you fit in perfectly.

You feel solid yet fluid. You feel lightheaded yet focused. So this is what contentment feels like, you think. You remind yourself you must do this more often.

You keep on walking and walking. Your breathing is becoming heavier and you can feel the muscles in your legs contracting and releasing with each step. You realize how good it feels to be active, how good it feels to be empty of worry, how good it feels to be alive.

You notice the smell of salt air. It reminds you of younger days, when a trip to the beach was so exciting.

You hear the subtle rhythm of the waves again just as a seagull calls in the distance. Your eyes look for the source of the sound and you notice an eagle soaring high above. It feels like you have been given special glasses to see the world with. I like these glasses, you think. They brighten everything around me. I no longer need those dark glasses I used to wear. An overwhelming feeling of joy and positivity is coursing through your entire being . . . body, mind, and spirit. You can see yourself on the beach. You are glowing with a spark that can never be put out. You can see that although you are alone on the beach, you are connected to everything around you . . . and words cannot capture how good it feels. You have lost all concept of time as you connect with a place that is beyond time. Eventually you realize you need to turn around. You do this without sadness or regret. You are just happy to have had this experience. As you start to walk back you notice your footprints in the sand. They are crisp and clear.

As you walk farther back along the beach, you notice other footprints. Where did they come from? you think. There has been no one on this beach the entire time I have been walking. The number of footprints grows and you find yourself starting to feel anxious and suffocated. As you get very close to your starting point, there are hundreds of footprints. There are so many that you can't see your footprints at all. The past hours are forgotten as you feel an overwhelming need to run.

How did you feel for the first part of this exercise (up to where you turned around)?

How did you feel at the end of this exercise? What do you think the ending represents?

What have you learned about your life and your footsteps?

The exercise above is about each of us having the awareness and courage to walk the footsteps that we know are the right footsteps for us. To follow our own way on the Dreaming Path. To do this, we need to have a strong sense of who we are. We need to have a strong sense of identity.

Given our identity is influenced by the way others see us, if we don't think about ourselves in a positive way (self-image, self-esteem, self-belief) we are continually vulnerable to living our lives in fear of other people's opinions and judgments. This can lead to us living our life continually trying to fit in. Doing this can prevent us from finding our true selves.

Prior to my breakdown my entire existence was about receiving validation from others. At no time was I able to leave my footprints in the sand. They were always subsumed by myriad other footprints. Thankfully my breakdown became a breakthrough as I discovered my sense of identity wasn't mine. After spending time walking Country with Elders, I learned a great deal about culture and, much to my surprise, about myself. I was thankfully then able to find the real me and walk my truth.

Many of us think we are living our lives in accordance with our truth but in fact we are not. We might not be aware of it, but in the daily chaos, under the pressure of managing competing demands for our time from those around us, and in the effort to satisfy the various expectations of those who matter to us, our focus on who we are and our story can become lost in the noise.

Do you think you are leaving clear, decisive, and purposeful footprints in the sand? (Others can join you, by the way, but they need to walk alongside you with respect, love, and humility.) Or are your footprints trampled over by a host of other people, leaving you feeling suffocated, invisible, irrelevant, unappreciated, directionless, and lost?

Now think about your identity. Is it owned by you or is it the product of other people's expectations, values, and rules? Are you walking the footsteps you want to walk? Is the story of your life a true reflection of who you are?

As you look, listen, learn, and grow, it is important to remember that part of your learning needs to be about you. Reflecting on what identity means to you, who you are, and what you are about is essential if you are to access your path of meaning, purpose, and contentment.

If each of us embraces the power of continuous learning, commits to truth-telling, and walks their footsteps in accordance with who they are deep inside, connectivity will increase as we individually and collectively grow. A better world will be the outcome of this renewal process.

Message 10

Look, listen, and learn. The world that surrounds you is your classroom.

Message 11

If you come to me knowing everything, I can teach you nothing. If you come to me knowing nothing, I can teach you everything.

Message 12

Knowledge is worth nothing if we don't share it.

Message 13

Seek truth in all that you do.

Message 14

Your life's journey has a purpose. It is special and individual—just like you. Respect it, honor it, own it, and walk it.

Chapter 5

Inspiration and Resilience

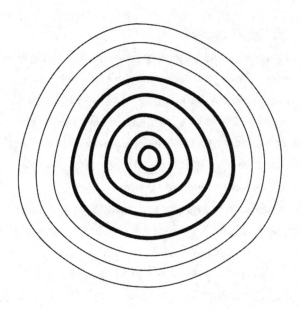

A long, long time ago, a young kangaroo named Wambuyn went down to the creek for a drink of water. The sun had only just come up and Kookaburra had only just started to laugh. He did this every morning to let everyone know it was time to get up and enjoy the day.

As Wambuyn was drinking, out of the corner of her eye she saw the glint of something small and dark disappear into the water. Being a very curious kangaroo, Wambuyn hopped over to the ripples to explore.

As she peered into the water she could see a small dark blur on the bottom of the creek. She was even more curious now, so she poked her head into the water to see better. When she did, she saw something she had never seen before. It was an animal with fur like hers, a beak like Garrangay the black duck, and a flat tail that looked out of place. What a strange-looking animal, she thought.

As she watched, she saw two beady eyes look up at her with fright. Wambuyn waved her paw in a friendly way, sat back down on the creek bank, and smiled.

After a very long time, a small furry head popped out of the water.

"Hello," said Wambuyn. "Don't be afraid. Why don't you come up and sit with me? I like to meet new friends."

The creature moved through the water as quickly as

Makurr the fish and in the blink of an eye was sitting next to Wambuyn. "I would like to have a friend," the creature said. "Hello. My name is Yapii."

Yapii and Wambuyn just sat there all morning having the biggest of yarns. By now, that old woman sun was high in the sky. Wambuyn looked up at the sun. "Oh my," she said. "I had better go. My family will be worried about me. I have never been away this long on my own." As she spoke, there was a loud crash and bang coming through the bushes. Yapii immediately jumped back into the water.

Waparr, the young kangaroo's father, appeared on the creek bank and looked very relieved. "Thank goodness I have found you, my daughter. You have never been away this long. Is everything OK?"

Wambuyn told her father how she had made a new friend and pointed to the dark blur in the water. Her father looked at her and smiled. "That is a platypus," he said. "You are very lucky to have a platypus as a friend. They are very shy and nervous. Hardly any of the animals have ever met one."

Waparr waved to Yapii and smiled. Yapii's small furry head popped out of the water again. "Hello there," Waparr said. "I am Wambuyn's father. I am so pleased to meet you. I can't wait to tell the rest of the animals that Wambuyn has a platypus as a friend."

"Really?" the platypus said. "You really think the rest of the animals would be interested?"

"Of course," the father said. "I know they would love to meet you." The three sat there and watched some dragonflies playing. "Hey. I have an idea," Wambuyn said to her father.

"Why don't we invite Yapii to come and meet everybody?"

"That's a great idea," he replied. "We can even have a corroboree in Yapii's honor."

Yapii jumped back into the water. Eventually he poked his head out. "I am sorry," he said. "I can't possibly leave the creek." He was shivering in fear.

"Don't be afraid," the father kangaroo said. "You are going to meet family. We are all one mob, you know. They will all be very excited."

"I have never left this place," the platypus said in a nervous voice. "I am so frightened. I would love to meet all of the animals I have seen come down to this creek, but I can't even think about it without feeling sick in my tummy."

"Yes, of course," said the father kangaroo. "I can see you are frightened. But think about it. If you let fear stop you doing something you would really like to do, you are letting it control your life. You are giving your power away to fear and missing out on something special."

Yapii crawled back onto the bank and lay on his back in the sunlight. "Hmm. You are right, but I just don't think I can do it."

"I understand," Waparr said. "We all get frightened sometimes."

"You are so big and strong. And you can move so fast. I can't see how you would be frightened of anything," Yapii said.

"Fear can show itself in many ways," Waparr said. "Over my life I have been frightened lots of times. When I was young, I was frightened of the dark. When I became an adult, I was frightened of failing to fulfill my responsibilities. When I became a father, I was frightened of not being a very good dad. And even now, sometimes I am frightened of letting people down."

"Wow," both Yapii and Wambuyn said at the same time.

"Being frightened is natural. Sometimes being frightened can save our lives. But most of the time, being frightened is our mind playing tricks on us. The secret is to not give in to fear when you know the fear isn't real. When we face fear, we are showing our courage."

Everything was quiet for a little while and then Yapii sat up. He looked different. "Thank you for your advice, Grandfather," he said. "If it is all right with you, I would very much like to come and meet all of my family. I don't know how brave I can be, but I will try my hardest."

Three days later, the animals held a very big corroboree for a very special guest. The guest was the strangest-looking animal. He had fur like a kangaroo, a beak like a black duck, and a flat tail that looked out of place. Although he was a bit shy to start with, his newfound family made him feel at home. He learned songs, he learned dance, and he heard many stories. He had the best night of his life.

What is your first thought when you wake up most mornings? Do you wake up with a feeling of excitement and enthusiasm for the day ahead? Or do you wake up feeling like you are a robot, doing the same thing over and over again?

To expect to be inspired as you wake up each day might seem

like the fanciful ramblings of a dreamer. Just the thought of waking up each day inspired might even bring on a feeling of exhaustion. But being inspired isn't about trying to pack a million things into one day. Being inspired is about embracing the sacredness of who we are and believing we were born for a purpose. We can't be happy or joyous all of the time, but we can certainly feel motivated and positive about what surrounds us at any moment in time. This doesn't require a lot of effort other than having the right attitude.

Feeling inspired rather than programmed or defeated makes it far easier to walk your footsteps and live a good story. By connecting with nature, fostering relationships, surrounding yourself with love, and viewing each day as an exciting chance to learn more, you are in a great headspace to bounce out of bed with a spring in your step.

There was a period of my life when darkness and anxiety were so consuming that I found it hard to get out of bed, let alone do it with a spring in my step. With professional help, I was able to realize I had given myself a number of negative labels that were not true. I discovered I was sabotaging my well-being through self-defeating, negative thoughts about myself and the world around me.

To turn this around, I learned how to look at myself and my story through a lens of love and friendship rather than condemnation and regret. By challenging how truthful my obstructive thought patterns were, I was able to discover the truth. My life, my story, was something I could feel good about. I was able to appreciate the power of my story and appreciate that everybody has a story that is remarkable and inspiring.

Exercise: Sharing Our Story

Sit down with a blank piece of paper. Think about your life story so far. Write down what you are happy with. Write down your regrets. Then put the piece of paper away for a while.

Contact two friends and ask them to do this Sharing Our Story exercise with you. You will need to meet with them face-to-face to carry out this exercise.

Explain to your friends that, when you give the go-ahead, one of them will have thirty seconds to tell the other their life story. After the thirty seconds has finished, the roles will reverse, with the other friend telling their life story for thirty seconds.

After they have done this, ask them to carry out the same activity, but this time, each person has thirty seconds to tell the other what they liked or found inspiring about their life story.

As both friends are doing the activities, observe their body language and the energy of the conversation.

At the end of the exercise, ask each person how they felt while they were doing it. You will more than likely discover that each person is surprised the other person found their story interesting, let alone inspiring.

This exercise aims to show you, as the facilitator, the importance of sharing story. If people can be inspired from thirty seconds of sharing story, imagine what is possible if we share story about ourselves for a longer amount of time and more often? This exercise also shows you how everyone has something remarkable in their story—including you.

Once you have completed the Sharing Our Story exercise, go

through your list of regrets and things you are happy with in your story so far. Is your list balanced? If it has more regrets than things you are happy about, are you being fair to yourself?

Pretend your life story belongs to your very best friend and you do the Sharing Our Story exercise with them, but for longer than thirty seconds. Which parts of their life story would you tell them inspired you? What feedback would you give them about their regrets?

Your friend's life story is precious. Yours is just as precious.

Being inspired is not easy, but it is not difficult either. If you really want to walk your footsteps, it is important to convince yourself that it is what you want, that it is worth it, and that you can do it. You need to believe in yourself and believe in your journey.

Sometimes it can be hard to believe. Our logical mind will tell us all sorts of things to try to protect us from disappointment and broken expectations. This makes sense—our mind wants to shield us from danger, both physical and mental. It is like an overzealous guard. By trying to care for us it can hold us back from doing things that are important to us.

Nurturing and growing our sense of optimism and hope is part of the antidote to the mind's tendency to overprotect and therefore undermine our belief in ourselves.

Think about children. We can learn a lot from children. Most children are examples of perpetual, inspired activity. They are specialists at harvesting the joy of the moment. They are wonderful role models and mentors of hope. The Easter Bunny, Santa Claus, dragons, unicorns, and fairies are not folklore to them. If you ask them what they want to be when they grow up, they will cheerfully offer up myriad thoughts without fear and without boundaries.

Is hope something you have in abundance? If it is, congratulate yourself and nurture it. If it isn't, ask yourself why not.

Some people might say they don't have time for such nonsense . . . that being an adult is about being practical and getting on with reality. I agree it's important to be grounded in our real lives as they are now, but I also argue it doesn't hurt to balance the scales with some hopes and dreams. Hopes and dreams are not impossibilities. If you are willing to learn and take small steps in the right direction, you will start to believe.

If we don't have hope in our story, then we find it hard to believe in our story. Without belief it is very easy for doubt to creep in to our thoughts and undermine our sense of purpose.

As we wake up each day, we never quite know what the next twenty-four hours has in store for us. This book gives you ways to see the positive that is all around you, but the reality is that some days are going to hold disappointment and unexpected events that might upset us or even make us feel like giving up. When we feel like this, it is OK to admit we don't feel OK. This is a time when relationships are important. It is a time to reach out for help or, on the flip side, for a friend to reach in and help. It is important that we open ourselves up to being helped so that the flame of hope can be relit.

The old saying "The longest journey starts with the first step" is an important call to action. Believing in yourself and knowing your journey is important will enable you to do extraordinary things and help others to do the same. But to take the first step of the journey requires hope.

Knowing you have the power within to undertake the journey is also important. Feeling empowered is an important component of feeling inspired. If you don't believe you have control in your life, it is very difficult to feel animated, excited, or energized about the day, the week, or the life ahead of you.

In the contemporary world, feeling in control can be a challenge given the many different people and processes dictating what we do every day. Things like work, work-related policies and procedures, government regulations, societal expectations, peer-group rules, and family responsibilities are all important realities we need to manage that, taken as a whole, can make us feel like we are caught in a maze. Yet work, government, society, peers, and family are not our jailers. The responsibility for breaking down the walls that confine us sits with ourselves. The means to freedom is also within us. This is a wonderful thing because we don't have to wait for anyone to break us out. True empowerment is not about blaming others; it is about understanding our inner potential and taking ownership of our actions.

Our Old People describe the process of empowered thinking as "connecting with your power."

In Aboriginal culture, we are taught that connecting to our power—that is, being empowered—is not a right we can claim. It is something we must learn and earn.

We earn our power through these choices:

- Looking and listening to our Elders, the Spirit Ancestors, the Father, and the Mother (builds our knowledge base, provides values to guide us).
- Looking and listening to our brothers and sisters in nature

(builds our knowledge base, gives us space to be ourselves and reflect).

- Following the Lore (provides us with boundaries and purpose).
- Being loving, humble, and respectful in all that we do (facilitates calm and connection).
- Believing in ourselves and our footsteps (gives us purpose and meaning).
- Accepting our responsibilities (gives us purpose and meaning).
- Knowing we are loved and do not have to prove ourselves to anybody (negates self-doubt and fear).
- Knowing that although there are rules we have to follow, we still have great flexibility and choice within the rules (provides us with space to consider options).

Taking ownership of your personal power is a liberating and rewarding experience. It is also a challenging and difficult journey to undertake. There are numerous Aboriginal sacred sites that teach us about power and being empowered.

It is important to understand that the significance of an Aboriginal site does not relate solely to how artistic or complex it looks. The importance of a site relates to the story and the learning that is within it.

Our people didn't create sites to make the bush look pretty. They didn't say, "Oh . . . this area looks a bit boring: let's do an artwork or engraving to give it some character." Our people created sites to teach us the Lore.

In traditional times an Aboriginal site was the responsibility of a number of people. There is the person who makes the site and there is the person who maintains the site. There is the story holder of the site, the holder of the song for the site, and the holder of the dance for the site.

When someone was taken there to learn about the site, all these people would be involved. This ensured the learning was right, and it ensured sharing and ensured unity.

Some people think that because Aboriginal people didn't have books, our knowledge system is somehow less sophisticated or effective than the Western system. This argument fails if you truly understand the Aboriginal learning system. Our Aboriginal sites are our books.

There are tens of thousands of sites across this continent that provide us with many libraries of knowledge. They are powerful educational resources for those who are willing to be a student. Although the sharing of knowledge through oral means was important, our Old People recorded our knowledge (history, value systems, and Lore) in many forms, including engravings, artwork, stone arrangements, carved trees, carved wood, and other items.

There is a place just north of Sydney from where you can see Mount Yengo. Biamii's footprints are in the stone, so you know it is a powerful place. There are also many engravings at this place that teach us many different things.

One engraving tells a story about a man who doesn't listen to his Elders and so does not grow in his learning and has no power. He is jealous of another man who has listened to his

Elders and is very powerful. The man with no knowledge or power is trying to steal the other man's knowledge and power.

The story teaches us to earn our power and not try to steal it from others. It also warns us that when we earn our power, we might attract lazy, egotistical, angry, jealous people who will try to hurt us and steal our power rather than earn their own.

Think about this story. Are you more like the figure who has earned his power or the figure who is jealous? What can you do to be more like the figure who has listened to his Elders? Think about your daily life. Are there any people in it who try to steal from you emotionally, spiritually, or intellectually? If there are, what do you need to do to stop this from happening?

Holding on to your power once you have earned it can be very challenging. The Old People warn us to not "give away our power or let people steal it from us." We can give away our power in a number of ways.

One way of losing or giving away your power is through fear. If you find yourself in a situation where you are genuinely in danger of being physically hurt, then fear is an expected and appropriate feeling. Much of the time, however, our fear is our mind telling us something negative will happen in the future.

We can become so consumed with the future that we are unable to live in the moment. We are like an insect caught in a web of apprehension, with a feeling that the spider is inevitably coming and the only outcome possible is a bad one.

When we do this, our life stories are put on hold. We become prisoners to our minds. Our self-talk is telling us things that aren't necessarily true, but we believe the chatter without questioning it.

The fear could be a fear of being ridiculed, a fear of rejection, a fear of losing something material, or a fear of losing your job. It makes no difference what the fear is about. Whatever the fear, if the anxiety is significant, your body will trigger a stress response sometimes called the fight, flight, freeze response, which is our natural reaction to stressful or dangerous situations. It's an instinctive survival response that instantly causes hormonal and physical changes and is the body's way of helping to protect itself from possible harm.

When the response is triggered, a number of chemicals are released into the blood, causing an increase in blood pressure, heart rate, and breathing. Other changes include an increase in blood sugar, alertness, muscle tension, and sweating; dilated pupils; pale and flushed skin; and trembling.

Problems can occur when the fight, flight, freeze response is triggered regularly. In the longer term, this can lead to:

- immune system disorders,
- digestive disorders,
- muscular problems,
- short-term memory loss,
- coronary disease,
- sleep problems, and
- depression.

Although these effects are a response to stress, it is important to note that stress is merely a trigger. How stress affects us depends on how we manage it. If we let worry take control, the anxiety it generates can be very debilitating to our peace of mind.

Over time the anxiety can feed fear and dread. When this happens, we are giving away our power and placing ourselves at risk in mind, body, and spirit.

When this happened to me, one of the biggest challenges I faced was trying to get adequate sleep. Numerous studies indicate that poor sleep can affect our judgment, perception, ability to learn, and ability to retain information. Poor sleep can also impact our performance in the workplace or behind the wheel, increase our risk of serious accident or injury, affect our mood, and create health problems such as heart disease, stroke, diabetes, infertility, and weight loss/gain.

A lack of sleep or poor sleep can exacerbate our anxiety and fear, further undermining our resilience. We can find ourselves spiraling downward into darkness, a place where we feel totally disempowered. The reality is, we have the power within to stop the spiral downward and ascend back into the light.

I have done both. When I had my breakdown and my life became a dark cloud of depression, I was owned by fear. Once I understood what was happening, I began the long process of reclaiming my power. Slowly and steadily I started to climb out of the darkness on a journey that did far more than heal me. Without noticing it, I eventually flowed past the point where the spiral down had started. I transitioned to a far better place. A place where the authentic me achieved a life of meaning and contentment beyond my hopes and dreams.

On my journey of healing and reclamation, in addition to recognizing my fears, I also acknowledged my unresolved anger. Although my anger was understandable, I realized I needed to let it go.

As I reviewed my life, I could see many things I had been giving my power away to.

It's pretty easy to know if you are giving away your power. For example, imagine you are playing one of those video games. They can be fun, so why not. The question is: "Are you in control of the video game or is it in control of you? Can you just put down that controller or does it tell you not to?" Your answer will tell you if you have given away your power.

Think about alcohol. Alcohol is not a bad thing. But depending on how you use it, it can be a bad thing. Are you drinking alcohol because you are happy? Or are you drinking alcohol to make you happy? If you answer yes to the first question, then that is OK. If you answer yes to the second question, then you have lost your power.

Mobile phones are another thing that people allow to steal their power. Can you leave your mobile phone in your pocket for an hour and not look at it? The world is going pretty badly when we are controlled by such a little thing.

You can give your power away in all sorts of ways—fear, anger, jealousy, grief, wanting to be liked, needing to be loved, avoiding conflict or negative feedback. You can give your power away by focusing too much on obtaining and holding on to material things (house, boat, car, clothes, money) and pursuing pleasure (gambling, alcohol, drugs, sex, food, or television).

It can also happen with religious icons, sporting heroes, and celebrities. People are put on a pedestal (they might not ask to be) and their every move copied and their every word treated as truth. A person who tries to copy an icon, hero, or celebrity is not accruing wisdom or becoming empowered (we can learn from other people but shouldn't try to be other people). They aren't leaving their own footprints in the sand.

There are two simple questions to help you identify whether you have given away your power. The first question is: "Am I in control of my actions/this thing or are my actions/this thing in control of me?" The second question is: "Is my behavior helping me walk my footsteps and to live a good story, or is it taking me away from these things?"

If your answer to question one is that you are not in control of your actions, then you have given away your power.

If your answer to question two is that your behavior is taking you away from living a good story, then you have given away your power.

Recognizing that you have given away your power is the first step to reclaiming it. The next step is to reflect on how you give your power away and why.

Exercise: Giving Away My Power

Listed below are many ways you can give away your power. Place a circle around any words that you think relate to you.

- Fear
- Avoiding negative feedback
- Anger
- Material things
- Jealousy
- Gambling

- Sadness
- Sex
- Wanting to be liked
- Alcohol
- Wanting to be loved
- Drugs
- Avoiding conflict
- Food
- Television
- Spirituality
- Popularity
- Wanting power
- Stress/anxiety
- Expectations
- Control
- Money
- Body
- Other

Look at the words you have circled and reflect on why you think you give your power away.

Write down any goals you would like to achieve relating to holding on to your power and the actions you need to take to achieve them.

Review your goals and actions every two months.

In identifying ways to become more empowered, it is important to recognize that some of your habits might have been in place for a very long time . . . so small steps in the right direction may be the best way to start this journey. Celebrate each step you take and remember to focus on the distance traveled as opposed to the distance between where you are and the destination.

If you are feeling disempowered, you might find it difficult to reflect on your situation and clearly identify the actions you need to take to turn things around. You might need a circuit breaker to give you some breathing space and blue sky.

When your head is too busy, a great way to create balance is to ground yourself. Any of the three Connecting with Place exercises in earlier chapters is perfect for this. If that approach doesn't suit, an alternative is to go outside, take off your shoes and socks, and rub your feet into the grass. As you do this, try to let go of any thoughts you might have and just focus on what your feet are feeling. Do it as often as you need to for as long as you like . . . and do it without any particular outcome in mind. Allow yourself to just be.

When we feel like we have given away our power, the Old People teach us not to berate ourselves. Making mistakes and drifting away from our path is how we learn. Traveling down dead-end roads and taking detours on our journey can be rich and rewarding experiences. Maybe a particular mistake we have made needed to happen in order for us to learn something important. Without this learning, we would not be able to achieve our life purpose. The mistake is therefore part of our journey.

Even if you don't believe in destiny, having an attitude that mistakes are useful learning opportunities is a far more productive way to view them than getting angry, labeling yourself stupid, or being down on yourself. Whenever things seem to be going wrong in my life, I reflect on what I can learn from the situation and trust that it is happening for a reason.

An example of this was when I left my role as CEO of New England TAFE in regional New South Wales to become CEO of the Aboriginal Housing Office in Sydney. Although I loved my TAFE job, I had a desire to work in a role more directly related to Aboriginal services, so I moved with the belief I would be able to do important things for Aboriginal people across the state. The role didn't work out, and within twelve months I found myself without a job. Despite feeling heartbreak that a seventeen-year career in public service was over, at a deeper level, a part of me trusted that things were happening for a reason.

After numerous unsuccessful job interviews over the following twelve months, my wife, Alison, and I decided to move back home to my traditional Country. Despite not having jobs lined up in the area, and despite having a very large mortgage, we both had faith that everything would work out. In the five years since the move, I have written several books, completed a PhD, and built both a successful consultancy business and a lifestyle of my choosing. Alison works part-time so she can enjoy more time in the garden. My Sydney career disaster has turned out to be a life-changing stroke of good fortune.

- Over the years, I have become quite adept at leveraging a crisis. My ability to accept my vulnerability, patiently float through my challenges, and come out the other side of a traumatic experience with learning and hope has helped me through a number of major storms in my life.
- A nervous breakdown . . . became a nervous breakthrough.

- My public-service career ending . . . meant my job no longer defines me.
- Watching my youngest brother, Billy, take his last breath at forty-six years of age on the saddest day of my life . . . was also a reminder to see the magic in every moment we are alive.
- Watching our son walk over to me with an almost severed hand from a table-saw accident . . . demonstrated to me the magnificence of the modern medical system.
- Seeing my mum's thumb detach from her hand in a tractor accident when I was the driver . . . showed me the humility of our Elders. On the way to the hospital, Mum said how thankful she was that it was her and not me or my dad.
- One of our children finding themself in crisis on the other side of the world prompted me to race to be by their side (which I was within twenty-four hours) . . . and allowed me to experience the kindness of a stranger who noticed me crying on the plane.

Being inspired is one thing. Staying inspired is another. Weathering the storm is a key part of this.

Exercise: The Storm

Imagine you are a tree on top of a mountain. You are not just any tree: you are the tallest tree in the forest. Your roots are deep and plentiful, anchoring you securely to the earth. Your branches and leaves are abundant, housing all manner of life. Your trunk is strong and broad. The many rings within your trunk are testimony to the many years you have stood on this mountain, proud and protective, watching over the brothers and sisters who are all around you, giving and receiving love each and every day.

How are you feeling?

You hear a distant rumble and look toward the western horizon. A storm is coming. A very big storm with dark clouds and a tinge of menacing green. Very quickly, almost too quickly, the distant rumble becomes louder and louder.

In what seems like the blink of an eye, the storm is upon you. The clouds are purple and black with rage. Lightning is arcing and forking from the heavens to the earth, and the noise is so loud you can feel it vibrating through you.

The wind is now smashing its way through the forest. You can see trees being uprooted and feel their pain as they crash to the ground. You watch with horror as other trees, trees larger and stronger than you, are snapped in half like small sticks.

How are you feeling?

The storm is almost upon you. You know your roots are deep, broad, and plentiful. You know you won't be uprooted. You also know your trunk is pliable, flexible, like rubber. If you need to, your branches can bend and touch the ground. You know that your ability to bend and flow with whatever happens around you means your trunk will never break.

How are you feeling?

Blue-sky days are there for us to enjoy. It is important to acknowledge and give thanks when life is humming along and all is good. No matter what we do, however, life will always deliver storms. We can't prevent them from coming but we can certainly expect them and learn how to manage them when they arrive at our doorstep.

In the exercise above, as the storm was about to strike, how did you feel and how did you face it? Did you grit your teeth and prepare for the battle with hope and trepidation? Did you worry about whether your trunk would break or major branches snap off?

Gritting your teeth and facing a storm with a stubborn determination to be an immovable object might be an option, but force meeting force in a violent collision can be a big risk. An alternative is to do the opposite. Instead of standing upright and immobile, maybe you can bend, flow, and move as best you can to accommodate what is happening around you. Your canopy nearly touches the ground and your trunk shows tremendous dexterity and elasticity, bending but not breaking. By being flexible, you are better able to weather the storm.

If we can face a storm with an attitude of curiosity and flexibility (underpinned by trust and belief), our fear can be contained. If we accept the storm and flow with it rather than fight it, our fear might even disappear. Instead of feeling anxious or frightened, we can also choose to see the storm as an opportunity—a chance to validate what we have learned in life as well as a chance to learn more.

We could start to see that storms can sometimes be a good thing. There might be some collateral damage but maybe those dead branches in our life needed to be pruned to enable new growth to emerge? The leaves that have been stripped from us will contribute to the ecosystem around us, providing humus and compost for other things to grow. Our small losses might contribute to the greater good of those around us.

Think about the storms you have encountered in your life. Do you think you fought them, ran from them, crumbled before them, or accepted them and managed them? Look back at some of the big crises in your life. What can you learn from them? What might you do differently the next time a storm invades your blue sky?

In Aboriginal spirituality, most storms in our life are welcomed. The Old People say, "The tests you are facing wouldn't be here if you weren't ready. So have faith in your teachers, have faith in your learning, and have faith in yourself."

Sometimes, however, there are storms that hit us with clouds that have no silver lining whatsoever. My brother's passing was one of those storms. These kinds of storms are catastrophic events that we would not wish on anyone. More often than not, however, the storms we face aren't this calamitous, and it's our reaction to them that is so damaging.

Anger, fear, anxiety, and sadness may still appear during these tough times, but if we manage our challenges with acceptance and understanding, their impact will be far less disruptive and sustained.

Having knowledge will prepare you to overcome any fear and anxiety you may face. That is how it was in traditional Aboriginal society. They could have had fear and anxiety over accessing food; however, their intimate knowledge of Country through song, dance, and story about their food sources meant they always knew that food would be there. For example, we knew the quandong tree would fruit every year and we knew when it would fruit because we had knowledge of our world.

With our knowledge of weather conditions, there were also times when we knew trees weren't going to fruit, and this might have created some anxiety among our people. But because our knowledge of Country told us this was going to happen, we were able to prepare for it and find a source of food somewhere else.

So staying in tune with the land and spirit, having intimate knowledge of land and spirit, and being connected to all things allowed us to deal with any fear and anxiety over what we knew might lie ahead.

In today's world, many live in fear of the climate crisis. If we know we have to do something about it, we can use our knowledge to understand what must be done and so replace our fear with action. But are we willing to do what must be done? Are we willing to change the values of our society to do it? Do we care about future generations or only about ourselves?

By continuously building our knowledge base, we are better able to understand whatever life throws at us. Once we have understanding, we are in a better position to respond to the situation. Sometimes we need to respond with clear and distinct action and sometimes the best response is to accept what is happening and go with the flow. When we go with the flow, we are choosing to take this action. We have decided to float along with the current until such time as we decide to act. This is different than being inactive due to fear. If we are caught in the fight, flight, freeze response, and the current begins to flow too quickly, we can feel like it is dragging us under—and we might feel too paralyzed to act. Although we might feel like we can do nothing about our situation, this is the time for us to go inward and find the courage to take action (with the help of others if needed).

Sometimes when a storm has passed in our life, we come through unscathed. Sometimes we might emerge from a storm with new growth. Sometimes, despite doing our best, we might find we have been injured or damaged. Our resilience, which is about how we bounce back from misfortune, change, or difficult life events, is critical when this happens.

To fully understand resilience, we first of all need to understand how it differs from endurance. If we are living our lives in a way where we push our minds and bodies to the limit, and soldier on no matter what is happening around us, then we are displaying incredible endurance. Endurance can be a lifesaver if you are lost in the wilderness without food, water, or warmth. In the modern world, endurance is almost essential in surviving the many competing demands we face. The definition of endurance is the ability to suffer something painful or difficult with patience. The key word in this definition is *suffer*. When we are demonstrating endurance, we are in a place of pain. This is not a good place to be in for an extended period of time.

Resilience, on the other hand, is about recovery. It is about coming through a challenging time rather than putting up with it. By taking care of ourselves physically, spiritually, and mentally, we move through the hardship and fully engage in the present with continued inspiration and belief in ourselves and our journey. Navigating the world can be hard at times. Without resilience, it can be even harder.

When life has knocked you down, don't compound the situation by knocking yourself and keeping yourself down. Try to review what has happened in a detached way. Ask yourself, "Why did this happen? How do I feel about what has happened? What do I choose to do about what has happened? What lessons can I learn? Do I need someone to help me deal with what has happened?"

When you are feeling beaten by life, it is more than likely that you won't feel particularly enthusiastic, optimistic, or hopeful about the present or future. This is completely understandable, given you have been through a traumatic experience, so don't pressure yourself to jump back into the water's current if you aren't ready. At the same time, you don't want to exile yourself from life any longer than you need to. Taking small steps to reconnect with day-to-day life and accepting that you might not feel on top of the world as you do this is a helpful approach in this kind of situation.

If you do the right things, the sun will break through the clouds of despair at some point in time. There is no need to seek the blue sky: it will show itself in due course.

Exercise: Resilience Habits

Listed below are a number of behaviors that can contribute to your ability to get back up when you have been knocked down. Rate yourself out of five for each behavior. Five means you are a master, and one means you aren't very strong in that behavior at this point in time.

- Being flexible
- Identifying what needs to be done in a given situation and taking action
- Learning lessons from things that don't go according to plan

- Connecting with others, including asking for help
- Doing something to relieve tension
- Believing in yourself
- Identifying and believing in your life purpose
- Practicing healthy habits that nurture your mind
- Practicing healthy habits that nurture your body
- Practicing healthy habits that nurture your spirit
- Laughing
- Being optimistic
- Spending time with nature
- Acknowledging self-defeating thoughts and letting them go (including resisting the temptation to awfulize)

What are the priority areas you need to work on?

What do you need to do?

How will you make sure you do what you need to do?

Being locked in a test of endurance will not have you waking up every morning with a feeling of excitement and enthusiasm for the day ahead, I see this lack of inspiration etched on far too many faces as I am out and about. I call these people "the grays."

The first time I noticed the prevalence of "the grays" was when I was in Sydney with Uncle Paul some years ago.

It was lunchtime and we were sitting in a food court not far away from Central Railway Station. As I casually observed all sorts of people rushing here and there, I noticed none of them were smiling. In fact, no one looked even remotely happy. They seemed to be coated in a bubble of gray.

As we sat down and looked at the food court dining options, I told Uncle Paul of the joy of banh mi (Vietnamese pork rolls). As we ate them, he agreed they were up there with one of his favorite foods, kangaroo tail baked in ashes. We were in a state of bliss. We were coated in bubbles of multihued iridescence. If you are currently living a life surrounded by color, you are well on your way to living a good story. This is your chance to spread the color so that those engulfed by gray can leave the endurance treadmill behind. This is your chance to use the inspiration you experience to inspire others—to help others find the magic in each day. By doing this you win, they win, their family wins, and their community wins.

In supporting others to find more color in their lives, we need to be careful to not cross the line from helping to saving. A "savior complex" is where an individual has an overpowering need to save people by fixing their problems. A savior complex is not helpful for the individuals we are trying to help as it can give them an excuse not to take responsibility for their own actions and undermine their motivation to address their problems.

When supporting someone, it is therefore important to:

- not offer advice without being asked,
- set boundaries,
- not attempt to convince them what they think or feel,
- not do the work for them,
- collaborate rather than solve, and
- listen.

Throughout my life, I have found Aboriginal Elders are very good at following these rules. They are always there to support but are careful to not cross the line and disempower the person they are trying to help.

Helping each other to live the best story possible is important. From an Aboriginal perspective, everything that exists—the planet, the flora, the fauna, and the people—are one connected organism. If something or someone suffers, then all of us are affected—true well-being cannot be achieved if all things aren't well. We are all in this together.

Each of us is sacred, each of us is special, and each of us has come into this world with a purpose. Part of that purpose is to embrace our unique spark in collaboration with the world's other 7.7 billion unique sparks, and make a shared commitment to caring for our place, caring for all things in our place, and caring for each other. By doing this, we start a process of renewal, a process that will create improved wellness for all things.

This should be our overarching inspiration as we wake up every morning.

What can you do to make this happen?

Message 15

Every day is an opportunity to be inspired and to inspire others.

Message 16

Feeling empowered requires you to believe in yourself and your journey. As you shine, don't let others dim your light: they can't if you don't let them.

Message 17

When the storms of life appear, face them with faith in what you have learned and what you will learn. Bend; don't break.

Message 18

Each time you overcome hardship, recognize and celebrate your courage and resilience.

Chapter 6

Being Present and Healing from the Past

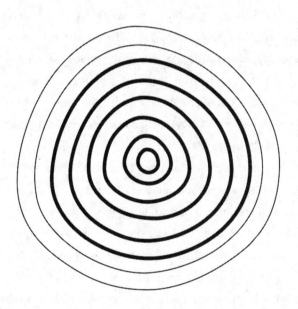

The emu chicks were up early this morning. Mother looked at their little faces and smiled. "Where will we go to find food today?" she asked.

"We can go back to where we were yesterday," one chick replied.

"Yeah. That was a good place," another chick said. "Let's go back there."

"Why?" said the mother. "We have already taken enough tucker from there. If we go back, it won't be the same as yesterday. And maybe that clever dingo will be waiting there to catch us. No, children. If we keep going back to the same place, we will get stuck in the past."

"I can see a mountain in the distance," another chick said. "Why don't we go there?"

"The mountains are far away," the mother replied. "We won't get there today. But we are here now." She slowly looked all around her and smiled. "This looks like a good place to gather bush tucker. Why don't we explore it?"

She looked down at the little heads nodding.

"We have to live in the now but also remember to bring the knowledge and the good memories of the past with us. So we can remember yesterday and smile but we must also remember to focus on today and find the smiles it will give us."

Mother looked toward the mountains. "Let's plan to take little steps toward the mountains. And each day as we gather our tucker, we will get a little closer to them. If we rush quickly to the mountains, we won't notice the beautiful things there are to see on the way."

The chicks were still nodding. They loved listening to the stories their mother told them.

"Let's stay in the now and connect with today. Tomorrow is another day and another story. We will connect with it when it happens."

Within minutes, the family found a tree covered in fruit. "This place is different from yesterday but it is still a very good place," a chick said as they all began to eat.

"It certainly is," another chick said. "I am so glad we are right here. This is the perfect place for us to be."

The mother emu sat and watched her children and smiled.

It was indeed the perfect place to be.

As I write, I am reflecting on the past two days of my life. The story of the last two days starts with a bigger story around a skin cancer (squamous cell carcinoma) located on my right calf that required surgical removal sixteen days ago. A three-millimeter spot on my skin turned into a fifty-millimeter incision requiring more than a dozen stitches externally plus internal suturing (a lesson to all about keeping an eye on your skin). The location of the wound required me to be stationary with my right leg raised for a period of two weeks.

Eleven days after the surgery, I noticed a dull cramp-like throb in my lower leg. I visited the doctor and was told that if it got any worse, to go and have my leg scanned. Fourteen days after the surgery I found myself in a medical imaging facility being told I had a very large (twenty-two-centimeter) deep vein thrombosis in four major veins.

Over the next five minutes, everything I thought and felt about the world was severely challenged. On the phone, my family doctor told me (in a voice that was a little bit ominous) to keep movement to a minimum until an ambulance arrived. She was fearful of a blood clot traveling to my heart. My heart started to race even faster when the doctor also told me she would contact the hospital emergency department to ensure they were ready for my arrival. Visions of television shows with critically ill patients being hurtled along hospital corridors flooded my mind.

My phone rang again. It was the ambulance service advising there would be a one-hour wait.

My doctor's response was one of disbelief. In her opinion, the wait placed me at an unacceptable risk. We agreed that my wife, Alison, should drive me to the local hospital, which was fifteen minutes away. Time slowed down and every traffic light seemed to turn red as we approached it. As each minute passed far too slowly, I did my best to not let my mind overwhelm me with negative thoughts and scenarios.

The care I received once I hobbled into Maitland Hospital Emergency was incredible. In the blink of an eye, I was in a bed being attended to by a doctor who was able to instantly put me at ease. After I returned home that night, I felt truly blessed to be alive. Facing my mortality in such an unexpected way had given me many things to think about.

In looking back at the last two days I learned:

- how important it is to listen to your body;
- how wonderful the medical system is;
- how blessed I am to have such an amazing partner;
- how unexpectedly precarious life can be;
- how critical my belief system is in times of crisis;
- how I have no regrets in my life;
- how important it is to stay present in times of acute stress, even when your brain is doing everything it can to take you elsewhere; and
- how important it is to see the magic and special moments in every day.

Many people fail to see the special moments in each day because they don't look for them. There are endless possible reasons for this, but a major culprit is our inclination to always be in a rush.

When you are next at a busy city railway station during peak hour, just stand still for a moment and watch what is happening around you. I bet you'll see lots of the following:

- people with their eyes glued to their phones, not daring to connect with each other
- people pushing and shouldering each other even before the train stops
- people trying to alight from the train being blocked by those trying to get on
- people squeezing themselves inside the closing doors, even though the train is obviously full

- people running to jump into the train as the doors are about to close, even though there is another coming in ten to fifteen minutes' time, or even less
- people inside the train placing bags next to them so others cannot sit down

When I watch these behaviors, I can't help wondering whether this is symbolic of these people's lives—constant rushing, running, pushing, shoving, isolating, not sharing, not caring, and placing other people's lives in danger?

If our Old People were to watch this scene, they would shake their heads. They would ask these sorts of questions:

- Why are people pushing and shoving?
- What is the rush?
- If this train is so important, why don't they come a little bit earlier?
- Is waiting less than ten minutes for another train so bad?
- Why don't people talk to each other?
- Why don't people share the seating that is there for everybody to use?

When we rush, we are at risk of triggering the fight, flight, freeze response outlined in the previous chapter. Unless there is a real and present danger, triggering this response isn't good for our mind, body, or spirit. In our daily lives, we can rush and trigger layer upon layer of anxiety or, alternatively, we can teach ourselves to slow down and embrace the moment, no matter what that involves. Which of the two behaviors has more likelihood of supporting our well-being? We can all argue that a one-off sprint to catch a train is not a major crime, but how often does this happen? Is rushing a habit?

In traditional Aboriginal life, there was little need to rush. Each day provided a multitude of opportunities to savor what was around you. Do you spend your day savoring what is around you . . . or does each day seem like a race against the clock?

In some ways, keeping an eye on the clock makes a lot of sense. Time is an instantly perishable resource that cannot be stored. It is the most precious of resources. When our time is up, all other resources (financial, human, natural, physical) are of no use to us. Given how precious our time is, it is understandable that we do as much as we can with it. The thing to contemplate is, when your time on this earth is almost finished and you look back at your life, how many of the things you rushed to do will you see as important or critical to your life story?

Our Old People teach us that the most important thing in our life is our story. Our story captures our actions from the past but it is built on what we do in the present. Upholding our responsibilities is an important part of what we do in the present. These responsibilities might include earning a living and servicing our basic needs for safety and survival, but they also include our responsibility to enjoy what surrounds us (the sound of a bird singing or the sight of a flower blossoming).

Aboriginal people have been doing this for more than 60,000 years. Mindfulness and being present in the moment are practiced when we walk Country, are practiced when we share story, and are practiced when we are doing what appears to be nothing.

The myth of Aboriginal people appearing to be doing nothing is captured in the word *walkabout*, which came into existence through non-Aboriginal people observing a behavior without understanding story. Had they learned our story, they would have realized that walking Country is an extremely purposeful activity that facilitates well-being of mind, body, and spirit.

The myth of Aboriginal people appearing to do nothing is also captured in the term "lazy Blacks." Had people understood our story, they would have realized that Aboriginal people carried out essential daily activities—such as food gathering, preparing meals, eating, and creating shelter—in a way that ensured there was always an abundance of time for sitting, teaching, and nurturing relationships. This was labeled as laziness by observers who didn't understand that Country gave you all you needed with minimal effort if you knew all about your Country.

These kinds of myths, which began hundreds of years ago, can become entrenched in society, creating stereotypes that exacerbate the social discomfort and trauma people might be living with. All of us need to be alert to commentary that contains preconceived ideas about characteristics and abilities of people who belong to a particular group. Otherwise, it is easy to subconsciously start to adopt similar ways of prejudiced thinking. Stereotyping and racial profiling fails to respect people's individuality and uniqueness, fans the flames of hatred, and generates disunity.

Often the stereotypes are hidden in seemingly neutral expressions. Phrases such as "Don't let the team down" and "Carry your weight" are examples of deficit thinking that have been used or paraphrased time and time again over the years. In this example, if we aren't careful, the underlying message of "Don't be lazy" can become an unhealthy mantra that drives people to work beyond what is reasonable.

Although work is an important part of our life, it is critical that it doesn't override other priorities. If we aren't disciplined about where work fits in to our life, it can undermine our well-being: Am I in control of it or is it in control of me? I learned this the hard way when, in my younger years, my inability to detach from my work led to chronic stress, sleep problems, difficulty concentrating, and family issues. I am by no means the only person who has suffered, and whose loved ones have suffered, from an unhealthy belief I need to "carry my weight" and "not let the team down." It is not something I would wish on anyone. In those years, my life had become totally out of balance.

Balance is a wonderful word and a call to arms for all of us to manage our needs, priorities, and responsibilities in a way that supports a state of personal equilibrium.

Nature, if left alone, will always find balance. Night and day ... the seasons ... birth and death ... everything is in harmony. Traditional Aboriginal society lived in harmony with the land. We ensured balance in all we did by looking at and listening to the land.

If we don't look and listen to the land, we create imbalance ... we create disharmony. If we don't look and listen to each other, we create imbalance ... we create disharmony. If we don't look and listen to ourselves, we create imbalance ... we create disharmony.

To live a good story we must find balance and create

harmony in our lives. We must find our truth and understand
what is important to us.

Look at the world. Is it in harmony or disharmony? Is it in
balance or imbalance? As Lore is forgotten, disharmony grows
and balance is lost.

There is no time like the present to restore it.

If our personal lives are not in balance, how can we expect our families to be in balance? How can we expect our communities to be in balance? How can we expect the world to be in balance?

It is very easy for our lives to become out of balance, and it can come about in an invisible way where we don't recognize that it has happened. Constantly pushing ourselves to accommodate workplace demands, spending most of our time trying to please others, telling ourselves it is only a temporary thing (but it becomes an entrenched habit), and measuring our success through how much wealth and how many material possessions we have accrued are all behaviors that can create imbalance.

In the workplace it is important to be able to monitor your workload and draw a line in the sand in terms of what is reasonable and what isn't. The pressure on workplaces to do more with less, combined with the fear of losing your job, can be a dangerous prescription.

Although it is a good thing to support others, it is important to do so for the right reasons. Doing it to please others means you are leaving yourself open to other people's judgments. The only person who you need to be answerable to is yourself. When you do things to please others you are giving your power away.

When we do something we know isn't good for us, sometimes we might say to ourselves it is a one-off as a way of convincing ourselves the behavior is OK. If it is a one-off action, then there is no problem, but if you are lying to yourself, there will be consequences. When you lie to yourself you aren't living your truth.

Having some money in the bank is obviously a good thing to have for peace of mind, but how much is enough? There is nothing wrong with spoiling ourselves every now and then by purchasing something nice. It could be a night out at a restaurant, or a clothing item, or something for the house, but it is important that we view our purchase as a bonus to our life rather than our primary source of joy. Having a large bank balance doesn't mean we are living a good story and doesn't mean we are on the Dreaming Path.

Although it is important to be vigilant with all of these potential triggers of life imbalance, consumerism warrants further attention given the seeds of this behavior are planted in our consciousness when we are so young. From when we first watch television, we are inundated with advertising and other messaging that tells us we need a certain toy or food to make us happy. As we get older the messaging broadens and sells us the notion that purchasing a particular car, house, item of clothing, look, vacation, or other product will bring us happiness. If we aren't careful, this messaging can:

• leave us ruminating on what we don't have rather than what we have,

- deceive us into wanting what we don't need,
- take us away from what is important to us at a deeper level,
- lead us to feeling envious of others who can afford what we can't afford,
- lead us to feel like failures if we can't get what we want, and
- create imbalance in our lives through overprioritization of money and material possessions.

Consumerism (which is not the same thing as trade) wasn't part of traditional Aboriginal culture. The consumerist mindset is part of the dominant Western culture we grow up in. Dominant culture defines the norms within a society, including language, religion, social values, and social customs, and can create pressure for us to conform to societal expectations rather than embrace our uniqueness.

When this happens we can feel conflicted. If the inner conflict isn't resolved we might start to question our original values and beliefs, and become confused about what our purpose in life is and who we are. We might feel we are going around in circles and start to wonder what life is all about. When this happens there is a real chance we have lost our way, lost our sense of purpose or lost our sense of connection. We are not on the Dreaming Path. Consumerism is only one of many ways that we can become lost. The important thing to believe is that when we are lost, there is always an opportunity to find our way home, to reconnect with our purpose.

Over the years, I have seen and met many people who were lost. Some had come from jail, some were from universities, and some were people in everyday life. But regardless of where they had come from, all had something missing in their lives that made them unhappy.

Some were drinking too much alcohol, some were taking drugs, some were angry, and some were sad. But once they were introduced to true connectedness through spirituality, once they took the time to connect back to nature and learned how all things in nature rely on each other, once they were sitting down hearing the land and feeling the land, once they heard the stories of how our spirits once walked Country, once they accepted that there is much more to life than just existing, once they realized that all we really need is to love this land and care for her and she will give us all we need, including shelter, food, happiness, and well-being, they were no longer lost.

When lost people listen, they realize the material world is full of wants that don't make us happy. Material possessions just make us want more and more. When we realize that all we need is the land and what she gives us, everything else becomes less important and less necessary. Then people become quite happy with what they have and they no longer feel empty, because their desire for more and more material possessions is lessened. Their happiness is based on contentment with what they have rather than what they want.

Thousands of Indigenous Nations have disappeared from the face of the earth because of the wants and greed of others.

Ask yourself, "Does one bathroom suffice or do I need three bathrooms in this house?" Can you tell me how having three bathrooms makes you happy? Why do you need five bedrooms when there are only two of you?

When you want more, you take more. When you take more, someone loses more. This has been the story of many Indigenous Nations of the world. Yet Indigenous people as a collective seem to be the only ones who care for and love our place the way it should be cared for and loved.

In the beginning, we were all Indigenous and we all loved the land and the land loved us. Throughout the ages, people have moved away from the land and stopped loving the land. They separated from the land by building villages, then cities, then supercities. Now the majority of the world's population doesn't feel the land, doesn't see the land, and doesn't connect with the land.

When the Europeans made contact with Indigenous cultures throughout North America, South America, and other places, it was a chance for them to learn and connect. Sadly, in the process, many Indigenous Nations disappeared forever. We must ensure their stories are not forgotten.

Consumerism, dominant culture, the workplace, wanting to be popular, and falling in love with money are all seductive ways to create imbalance in our lives. Another way to give our power away is to focus too much on the past or the future.

When we focus too much on the past, we can become stuck in a time warp of our own making. Whether we are reliving happy memories or unhappy memories, living in the past is a sign that we aren't that happy with our life at present. We are using the past to avoid our responsibilities to the now. Living our life in the past is a bit like navigating a car down the highway by looking in the rearview mirror. At some point, the car will veer off the road.

Planning for the future is a healthy and motivating thing to do but, given that the future doesn't exist and tomorrow is not guaranteed, it is important to do so in a balanced way. If we aren't careful, thinking too much about the future can lead to "when-then" thinking. Examples of when-then thinking are captured in statements such as these:

- When I get my new video game—then I won't be so bored.
- When I get my new car—then I will know I have made it.
- When I get a house on the beach—then I can invite people over.
- When I lose fifteen kilograms of weight—then I will feel good about myself.
- When I knock off today—then I can finally get away from all this stress.
- When my holidays come—then I can go to a place with no phone signal and have some peace and quiet.
- When I retire—then I can do what I want with my life.

The problem with when-then thinking is it takes us away from engaging in the joy that can be found in the present. Resisting the temptation to focus too much on future happiness is hard but important if you want to achieve a state of improved well-being. Focusing too much on the future, including when-then thinking, is a bit like driving a car down the highway by looking five hundred meters ahead. At some point the car will veer off the road.

The way to stay on the road, of course, is to focus on the road immediately in front of you. To focus on the present.

Here are some of the many benefits of living in the present:

- relieves stress
- increases focus
- improves emotion regulation
- increases emotional intelligence
- increases empathy and gratitude
- increases resilience
- improves creativity
- lessens negative feelings
- lessens the risk of heart disease
- lowers blood pressure
- reduces chronic pain
- improves sleep
- alleviates gastrointestinal problems

These benefits provide a compelling case for making "being present" a high priority in your life. Acknowledging the benefits of being present (mindful) is the first step to anchoring yourself in the now and letting go of the habit of thinking too much about the past and future.

By giving yourself permission to focus on you and allocating the time to carry out mindfulness exercises regularly, you might find you are more able to stop pressuring yourself to be continually busy. This might feel strange at first, but resist the temptation to slip back into the bad old habits of rushing. Constantly remind yourself of the benefits if you need to. You are worth it!

Ever since I became a Lore Man, I have practiced being in the now almost continuously, to the point it has become a habit for me. There are times, of course, in my present professional and nonprofessional life where I reflect on the past, think about the future, and even plan for the future, but I do so without taking away from my connection to the present.

How well do you connect with your surroundings? When did you last notice how good it feels to have sunlight on your skin? When did you last notice the colors of a sunset? When did you last notice the sound of laughter? When did you last notice the taste of butter on corn? When did you last notice the smell of freshly cut grass? Connecting with our senses and connecting with what is around us helps us to be present.

To help me create the habit of being in the present, I developed what I call the T.E.N.S.E. routine. The letters in the acronym T.E.N.S.E. prompt you to connect with your senses as follows:

	Sense	What good things have I . . .
T	Tongue	tasted today?
E	Eyes	seen today?
N	Nose	smelled today?
S	Skin	felt today?
E	Ears	heard today?

If you commit yourself to ten minutes of the T.E.N.S.E. routine toward the end of every day (which equates to two minutes for each sense), you will be amazed at how much less tense you feel. If you are having problems going to sleep at night, or getting back to sleep when you wake up, T.E.N.S.E. might give you some welcome relief.

Exercise: T.E.N.S.E. Yourself to Sleep

Try to memorize the routine below. Use it whenever you are having problems going to sleep or getting back to sleep.

Go back through your day.

From when you awoke this morning to when you got into bed, think of each letter and what it stands for.

T (Tongue)—Think of all the good things you have tasted today.

It might be the taste of toast, butter, and jam you had for breakfast. It might be the taste of cereal and the taste of milk.

Calmly float through the rest of your day remembering all the wonderful tastes you have enjoyed.

E (Eyes)—Think of all the good things you have seen today.

It might have been your partner sleeping when you first woke up. It might have been the sun streaming through a window.

Calmly move through the day noting various random things you saw that made you smile.

N (Nose)—Think of all the good things you have smelled today.

It might be your first coffee of the day. It might be the air when you first went outside.

Calmly move through the day remembering things that had an aroma that you enjoyed.

S (Skin)—Think of all the good things you have felt on your skin today.

It might be hot water in the shower. It might have been the sun, or a breeze, or a raindrop on your face.

Calmly move through the day remembering things that you have felt on your skin that felt great.

E (Ears)—Think of all the good things you have heard today.

It might be the alarm letting you know you are alive. It might be music on your way to work.

Calmly move through the day remembering things you have heard that made you feel happy.

As you work through the various senses, you might be pleasantly surprised to find out the next morning you didn't get to finish the T.E.N.S.E. routine. It is unusual for a process to be judged a big success if you didn't finish it, but that is the case in this instance.

Much like the Gratitude Diary exercise and the 10/10 Moments exercise, if you continually practice the T.E.N.S.E. exercise, you will start noticing positive things in your life as they happen.

You will discover that many of the highlights of each day are harvested rather than manufactured. So it is good to know you don't really have to do much other than notice what's happening around you to start improving your well-being.

Noticing what is around you, however, can be harder than it sounds. For instance, when you first try looking with awareness, the mind has a tendency to respond to that quietness as if it is boredom—and try to fix the problem by entertaining and distracting you. It is used to managing a constant influx of important and unimportant messages and triggers, and may warn you something isn't quite right if this work rate isn't maintained. But if you sit still often enough and long enough, that "monkey mind" chatter will ease off and your surroundings will start to spring to life.

Let's imagine you have found a quiet place to sit in the bush. If you patiently allow the boredom to come and go, you might start noticing how individual each tree is—how each tree moves differently in the breeze; how each tree has its own color, size, and shape; and, if you reach out with your spirit, you might even find each tree has a unique personality.

You might notice a bird flitting here and there and ask yourself whether it has been there this entire time. Then you might notice other birds. Don't be surprised if some of them are looking at you with interest. You might also surprise yourself by noticing you can hear silence and how good it sounds.

You might look to the ground and notice a variety of insects. As you watch them you might start reflecting on why they are moving in various directions. You might watch an ant and ask yourself, Has it a plan? How does it know its way home? Does it get stressed or bored like I do? And then you might realize you don't need any answers and gently let the thoughts go.

You might notice the clouds and remember how you used to love looking at their shapes when you were a kid. You might notice how the bush changes color when the clouds cover the sun. If you stay there for a while, you might notice how the shadows move during the course of the day and how moss grows on a certain side of a tree.

If you stay late, you might notice how the bush transitions from afternoon to evening to night. You might decide to go for a short stroll in the darkness and be surprised how much you can see, even when there is little moonlight. If you look up, you might notice how bright the stars are, how many there are, how they are different colors and sizes, and how they seem to sparkle. You might notice the constellations and how they move through the night, providing points to navigate by. You might also notice the darkness between the stars. In these dark spaces sit many stories. Sometimes it is what you can't see that has the most value.

By actively looking and listening, you will notice a great deal and possibly achieve some surprising insights. You might discover patience, beauty, persistence, hope, trust, change, diversity, unity, and who knows what else. All this comes through letting go of the chatter of the mind and flowing with what is around you in the now.

If you do this regularly, you will start building relationships with what is around you and begin to understand the interconnectedness of all things. Once you are well practiced, you will find that you can do this anywhere—in a shopping center, in a park, on a street, sitting in your front yard, or in your backyard. As long as you aren't intruding on people's privacy, watching the world go by can be a very rewarding experience.

Exercise: Watching the World Go By

Over the next few days, plan a ten- to fifteen-minute break.

Find somewhere you can sit comfortably and safely in the open air and not be interrupted.

Take a deep breath in through your nose, hold it for a couple of seconds, and then let it out slowly through your mouth. Do this a few times and notice your tummy rise and fall with life-giving air.

Let whatever thoughts you have flow in and out without any effort. Don't try to hold on to them and don't worry about pushing them away. Just acknowledge them and then let them go.

When you are ready, look at things as if you are from another planet. Look in a soft, patient, curious, calm, and detached way. As you focus on a particular object, look at it in detail in an unhurried way and . . . when you are ready . . . move on to something else. You aren't trying to look at everything that is around you; you are more interested in noticing just a couple of things but in great detail.

After you have completed about three minutes of looking, close your eyes and listen. Listen as if you are from another planet. Listen to sounds close to you, listen to sounds far away. Do this for about three minutes without judgment.

After you have completed around six to seven minutes of looking and listening, reflect on what you have seen and heard. Were there any surprises? Did you notice things you hadn't noticed before? How do you feel? Did you find that thoughts of your day so far kept on intruding or did you find that you escaped that world for a little while? Did you gain any insights? Are you going to do this exercise again?

The more you do this exercise, the better you will become at connecting with the present.

Although it is important to live in the present and be aware that it isn't good for you to live in the past, that doesn't mean we should forget the past. Most of us have events and experiences that have been difficult, sad, or traumatic. Sometimes we are told the best way to deal with these things is to forget about them and move on, but that doesn't necessarily help us.

Your past is important. If you don't know your past, if you don't know your story, if you don't know where you come from, then you will be sitting in the present moment lost.

A lot of people say to me, "Ooh, look. The trouble with you Aboriginal people is you won't forget the past. You won't forget about what has happened to you." They say, "Forget about the atrocities that happened to you and move on."

A lot of people think that the future is all that matters. But how can you move forward into the future if you don't know where you have come from? What are you taking with you into the future if you aren't taking the past with you? The past is all you have.

Imagine if you were somewhere other than here. You were somewhere else and I clicked my fingers and brought you to a place and you didn't know how you got there, you just appeared there. How would you feel? You would feel lost. You would feel confused. You would feel frightened because a part of your story is missing.

And if at the end of the day, someone said, "Why don't you go home?" you wouldn't be able to because you don't know how you got to where you are in the first place. So when someone says, "Go home," you say, "I don't know how to."

If you knew about your past, that would enable you to go back to where you came from, and that's really important. People say, "You can't change the past." No, you can't change the past, but you can look back to where you were in the past and know where you have come from. You have a place to go back to.

So I can always go back, even though I might choose to move forward. I have that choice. But if I don't have that story of my past, I can't go back, and if there are things from the past hurting me, holding me down, affecting my self-esteem, I might end up being angry or I might end up being sad. I can't change my past but I can address it. To address it, I can look back at the past and say, "Why am I feeling this way? How can I address what happened to me that made me feel this way?"

It is only by having the ability to go back and look at the past that I am able to address what has happened. By addressing the past, I can change my present situation. So you have to know your story. So many Aboriginal people don't know their story because their past has been taken away from them and not even acknowledged.

Government Acts, the Stolen Generation, the removal of people from Country, massacres of the Old People, and our people dying of diseases took away the past for so many of our people. So our people are trying to operate in the present moment without any story, without any connection to the past. There are lots of people who are like orphans. Who are trying to live in the present moment with no connection to the past. They are like children. All lost. The reason Aboriginal people have more drug addiction, more suicide, and more alcoholism is because many of our people are disconnected.

Only by addressing their story can you really place them in a better position.

Without our past, we have no story. If we dismiss our past, a part of us will be missing. We will have lost our foundation and the learning it contains.

In traditional times, Aboriginal people went through hard times and went through good times just like we do today. As a group, Aboriginal people had to manage droughts, floods, and other changes in the natural environment. They were able to respond to the challenges by learning from the past. This learning provided an understanding of nature and how to flow with nature rather than fight it or try to control it.

In our stories from the past, hard times came upon us when we stopped carrying out the Lore. Some of our stories talk about big droughts and big floods that happened when people thought they were above the Lore. From these stories we were reminded of the importance of following the Lore.

The stories told us how to deal with the hardships when they came: for instance, where to find water when the droughts come. There is a story that tells us the water is sometimes not in the river but in the roots of the trees or sometimes in the mouths of frogs.

Since the creation, all native plants and animals have learned to adapt to the climate they are in. For Aboriginal people, although things might have been hard at times, they were never life-threatening.

The reason they were never life-threatening was because the people who came before them faced the same hard times and learned from those hard times and passed that knowledge on to us. If we had rejected the knowledge of the past, we would have perished. The same thing will happen to you if you keep rejecting the knowledge of the past.

From a global perspective, there are many lessons to be learned from the many hardships humanity has endured. In the last few years, the world has been subjected to wars, terrorist attacks, volcanic eruptions, tsunamis, cyclones, earthquakes, droughts, floods, bushfires, economic crashes, and pandemics. It is important that we learn from such tragedies. What is even more important is that we share that learning so we are better able to avoid or manage similar occurrences in the future.

From an individual perspective, our stories might also include significant hardship. Sometimes the trauma of our past can create chains that imprison us. Trauma is an unpleasant experience, but if it is affecting our present, it is something we have to face. By understanding the source of our pain, we can take action to break the chains and allow ourselves to bathe in freedom, peace, and lightness of spirit. If the pain is significant, we might need to seek professional guidance to help us.

You have only one story and it is important for you to acknowledge and embrace all parts of it—the good, the bad, and the ugly. Your past is part of who you are. By making friends with it, by looking at it without judgment, by understanding that your past has been your path to the present, you will find the need, determination, and strength to go back and identify those things that you need to address.

Once you do this, you might find that, instead of harboring regret for perceived failings, you might be able to find acceptance for what happened and free yourself from the confines of self-judgment.

Sometimes our past can give us learning we can use in the now. I know that from my hard times, I have been able to improve my life skills in a number of ways. The storms of the past have given me:

- increased resilience,
- greater discipline,
- increased comfort with feeling vulnerable,
- increased empathy for others,
- the ability to ask for help,
- the ability to help others,
- courage and fearlessness,
- an increased ability to problem-solve,
- increased patience,
- a greater ability to be present,
- the ability to actively listen,
- an increased ability to reflect on my life,
- a clearer understanding of my life purpose,
- a trust that everything is going to work out as it should, and
- an increased ability to let negative thoughts go.

If you look back at your life, you might find the hard times have helped you in some of these areas as well. The list of learning and knowledge the school of hard knocks gives us is endless. To harvest the learning this school provides, it is important to be honest about our past and learn from our mistakes. When looking at our past, it is also important to celebrate the good parts of our journey so far (if you find it hard to identify any good parts, the Sharing Our Story exercise in Chapter 5 will help). By addressing, learning from, and celebrating your past, you will be in a stronger position to reflect on your present and assess whether you are living your truth. After you do this, you are better able to examine all you've experienced and learned so you can ensure that you continue living your truth and leaving your footprints in the sand.

This begs two obvious questions: "How do I know I am living my truth? How do I know I am leaving my footprints in the sand?"

The Old People answer these questions very simply. They would say, "Connect with your belly and see what it tells you. If it feels warm and happy, then you are. If it feels cold and not right, then you aren't."

If you are more comfortable with analytical and cognitive approaches to problem-solving, you might ask yourself, "Do I feel like I am doing what I am meant to be doing with my life?" And then you could write down a response that captures how you feel. A second question might be, "Do I feel I am living . . . or do I feel I am just existing?" Again, you could write down a response so you have something to reflect on.

We all encounter difficulties and challenges in our lives of course, but if it seems that your life is a never-ending series of dramas and struggles, it could be a sign that you are not living your truth, that you are not on the Dreaming Path and not fulfilling your life purpose.

If your answers suggest you aren't living your truth, you may find you need to contemplate making changes in your life. Many people fear change, as it generates uncertainty and a potential loss of control. Uncertainty pushes us out of our comfort zones and can create inner resistance. Our fear of change can be so pervasive that we put up with being unhappy rather than risk the unknown (for many people, routine provides comfort). Breaking the status quo of certainty can therefore be very threatening. Sometimes people are just happy to go around in circles.

Often people won't change until they are at a point in their lives where they feel like or they actually are going to hit rock bottom. This is a bit like going to the doctor when you have pneumonia rather than when you had a runny nose. Prevention is always better than the cure.

Aboriginal people have always been harvesters of change. We knew the many seasons and looked forward to them. We looked forward to them because we knew the land, could read the land, and knew what was coming. We knew we needed to go to different places at different times, and we knew when we got there we would have different foods to eat, different sites to visit, different ceremonies to perform, and different stories to share. Sometimes there would be gatherings of different people to meet.

For us, change was never uncertain and never fearful. We knew where the path would take us. Change is part of the cycle of life. It is an important part of renewal. If we become set in our ways and we don't flow with what is around us, we can become stuck in the past and left behind. If that happens, how can we stay connected? Change is part of flow. Flow is part of connectedness. Connectedness is the path to contentment.

You can use your past and what you have learned from your story so far to ensure that the rest of your life, the next chapters of your story, are owned by you and are written by you. This is an exciting prospect.

For most of us, writing a book isn't easy. We might have some good ideas, but forming the ideas into a readable narrative can be daunting. Most of us wouldn't feel embarrassed about getting some help to do this.

Writing the story of your life is no different. Getting some support, advice, help, and guidance can be a great way to get your story up and running. There is nothing to be embarrassed about. Remember, however, you need to be patient. The story won't be written overnight. There will be times when the words cascade forth and times when they will be hard to come by.

There will be rewrites of pages and pages thrown out. Be kind to yourself when this happens; it is all part of the creative process.

Exercise: Making a Change

Identify something in your life you are unhappy with that you would like to change.

Try to choose a change that is reasonably important but achievable for you. You want to do something that isn't too big. Big things can come later. (If you are having difficulty choosing, go back to the Building Self-Respect exercise in Chapter 3. There might be something there that appeals.)

Write down all the reasons you need to make this change in your life. Once you have finished, read through them slowly. What you have listed is your storyline for change. It is your evidence base. It will be your motivation to continue should you ever feel like giving up. You now have the why.

Write down all the things you need to do to make the change happen. You now have the how.

Write down the things that might stop you from making the change. Go back over them and identify how you will manage these things so they won't get in your way. You now have your contingency plan.

Close your eyes and imagine your life when the change is in place. Watch yourself in the situations where the change is evident. How do you look? Open your eyes.

How do you feel?

Now put your actions in motion.

Once you have been successful in making the change, make sure you take the time to congratulate yourself and celebrate your achievement. You have earned it.

You are now ready to pick another change or changes you would like to make. By empowering yourself to make change you are increasing your ability to make choices in your life. Increased choice means increased opportunity to walk your footsteps and achieve increased contentment and well-being.

Think of a time in your past when you had your heart set on doing something challenging and eventually did it. It might have been learning to play a musical instrument or cook or build or sew or paint. It might have been losing weight or growing your own vegetables. It might have been getting your driver's license. Did you become a master of this discipline in twenty-four hours? Of course not. You needed to learn at your own pace in a way that suited you. Practice . . . fail . . . get back up . . . practice some more . . . improve . . . learn . . . seek advice . . . nearly give up . . . keep on trying . . . improve some more . . . don't give up . . . get there . . . celebrate. This is often how the path unfolds, but it is worth it.

In following this path, remember that it must connect to your truth and that in Aboriginal spirituality your path sits within an overarching path, the Dreaming Path. When our path and the Dreaming Path are in alignment, we are well. When they aren't, we can become sick.

The Ngurrampaa explains how things came to be and your relationship and responsibility to all things. Your connection to the Dreaming Path is about how you carry out these responsibilities each day. How you are following the Lore. It is about learning from the past so you can do the right thing in the present. If you are not following the Dreaming Path you can become sick. If you become sick you cannot carry out your responsibilities. As I look around me, I see many people who are sick. As I look around the world, I see many places that are sick. The earth itself is sick.

Because of our holistic approach to well-being and our intimate knowledge of our food and medicine sources, there was very little illness in traditional Aboriginal times. The people were well and the earth was well.

If people did get sick from an unknown sickness, there were Old Men and Women who were faith and spiritual healers who could lay their hands on you and heal you. We believe that some illnesses are caused by a sickness in our spirit. Given the spirits

*that are around us, by doing a clearing ceremony, the sick
person can be healed this way as well.*

*All things play a part in the healing of a person, not just a
pill. As a result of living a natural lifestyle and being connected
with spirit and Country, many of our people lived to be very old.
Much older than our people today.*

*As I look around me, I see many people who have sickness in
their spirit. This is another kind of pandemic placing the world
at peril. But for many reasons, most people do not see it or
want to see it. If they don't see it, how can they acknowledge it?
If they don't acknowledge it, how can they cure it?*

Without truth, healing cannot take place.

When we go through any kind of hurt, injury, or trauma,
we need to heal. Healing is a process that has been recognized
throughout history and throughout different cultures. In its sim-
plest sense, healing is the process of enabling someone to become
healthy again. Being healthy means different things to different
people and cultures, but in a holistic sense, to achieve a state of
well-being, there are four pillars that must be firm:

- emotional (being mindful, managing stress, positivity,
  learning);
- social (connectedness, relationships, community);
- spiritual (time in nature, meditation, belief, faith); and
- physical (sleep, diet, exercise, not smoking).

If you reflect on traditional Aboriginal life, you will see that
the four pillars and the key activities within them were integrated

into daily activities. This is why the majority of Aboriginal people lived long and contented lives.

Most of us recognize the importance of doctors, psychologists, psychiatrists, and other health professionals in facilitating the healing process. The Western medical system is something we can all be thankful for. At the same time, alternative health practices can sometimes complement the Western system and achieve even more outstanding results (traditional Aboriginal healers, sometimes called Ngangkari, are an example).

Your story is unique, as are you. Your pathway to well-being will be unique as well. Given the healing journey is such an individual and complex one, it is important to reflect on what "healing" means to you (possibly with the help of professionals) so you can undertake a therapeutic process that addresses the past and allows you to fully embrace the present in a positive and healthy way.

From an Aboriginal perspective, healing involves connecting with Country, connecting with spirit, connecting with Lore, and reflecting on the many themes covered in this book (story, relationships, unity, sharing, love, respect, gratitude, humility, learning, truth, inspiration resilience, and being present). There are two additional elements of traditional Aboriginal society also worth reflecting on.

The first element is laughter.

If you ever get a chance to watch archival footage of the Old People going about their daily life, you will notice they laugh a lot. The old saying "laughter is the best medicine" is very wise advice.

Think about your favorite comedian or favorite television or movie comedy. How do you feel when you watch it? Can you remember a time when you laughed so much that tears streamed down your face? How good does it feel?

For traditional Aboriginal people, laughter was an important part of life. Laughter facilitated connection, nurtured relationships, and was used by the Old People as a part of the teaching process.

> Every night, as part of their entertainment, Aboriginal people would act out something funny that happened during the day so everybody who wasn't there could experience it as well, and from this playacting everybody knew what happened that day and could all laugh together.
>
> In our daily life, as the Elders were teaching us, they were also teasing us with little stories and jokes, teaching us to laugh rather than be upset at the world of silly people.

Laughter is still very much used today by Aboriginal people to connect and sustain relationships. For many Aboriginal people, laughter is also used as a means of coping with the pain and suffering they have endured in their lives since occupation in the late 1700s.

Using laughter as a remedy for emotional pain and suffering is not uncommon in today's world, as it is thought to give us numerous benefits. Laughter:

- boosts immunity;
- exercises diaphragm, abdominals, and shoulders;
- lowers stress hormones;

- burns calories;
- decreases pain;
- reduces blood pressure;
- relaxes our muscles;
- improves breathing;
- prevents heart disease;
- improves our mood;
- eases anxiety, tension, and stress;
- boosts confidence;
- strengthens resilience;
- gives us a distraction;
- changes perspectives;
- strengthens relationships;
- promotes goodwill;
- enhances teamwork and group bonding; and
- attracts others to us.

The power of laughter is therefore well worth exploring on our journey toward improved well-being.

Before my breakdown, I was seen by many as the life of the party and a happy-go-lucky person. This observation was partly accurate, but much of my comic bravado was cloaked by major self-doubt and insecurity. My "smiley mask" was something I often wore so people would like me. I was addicted to other people's approval. I needed it in order to feel worthwhile.

So when you find yourself laughing, it is sometimes beneficial to think about the reason you are laughing. Are you laughing to fit in? If so, you might need to think about why. Are you laughing at someone else? If you are, is this being fair and respectful to that person? If it isn't, you might need to think about why. Are you laughing because you are happy? If so, congratulations. Keep it up. Laughing is infectious. Hopefully you can be a catalyst to others.

In the midst of my breakdown, I remember sitting outside my parents' house one day and hearing a strange sound I didn't immediately recognize. After a few seconds of searching, I realized the strange sound was laughter. It was, in fact, my laughter. I hadn't laughed for so long, I had forgotten what it sounded like. As my healing journey progressed, I laughed more often. I laugh a lot these days and, even better, I laugh for the right reasons.

How often do you laugh? Do you laugh enough? Do you laugh at yourself when you do something silly or do you get angry? Would other people describe you as funny or the life of the party? If so, is this an accurate picture of who you really are? If you don't think you laugh enough in life, make it a regular thing by setting aside a time regularly to laugh. This might sound contrived, but being organized will help you make sure it happens. You might choose to laugh with some friends or by yourself. You might laugh about something funny that has happened to you, watch a funny movie, watch a funny television show, read a funny book, or see a comedian live. This benefits you whether your laughter is genuine or pretend.

The second element to reflect on in terms of healing and being present is loss.

Of all the traumas that can befall us, the feeling of loss would have to be one of the most painful. When we suffer profound loss, we may rightfully need to press the pause button on life, but at some point, we will need to press play again . . . we will need to address how we are feeling so our life is not put on permanent hold.

Losses can occur in all aspects of our life. The loss of a loved one can obviously be a terrible, painful, and crippling experience. There are also numerous other experiences that can be traumatic for us:

- loss of health
- loss of love
- loss of employment
- loss of a house
- loss of confidence
- loss of freedom
- loss of peace of mind
- loss of faith
- loss of financial security

Our reaction to loss can range from mild annoyance to being overwhelmed and unable to breathe. When loss is substantial, it is important to grieve.

Learning about grief, including the interwoven stages you will pass through and revisit, can help you understand and accept how you are feeling at any moment in time, and facilitate the healing process. Due to the profound and traumatic nature of loss, it is best to gain this understanding through a recognized and qualified expert in this field.

If, in your grief, the thought of having to converse with other people is all too much, a stepping stone of renewal can be to spend time connecting with the natural environment. Finding a place outside where you can reconnect with your senses and nature in a way that feels right, feels safe, and happens at a pace you choose can provide the nurture you need without being too confronting.

From these initial steps, you can build on the healing that nature provides and gently reengage with life in a way that respects your story and helps you find peace. This can include accessing professional support, as mentioned above, to help you better understand what you are going through. When sharing your grief with someone else, it is important to ensure you are doing so with the right person . . . so it is perfectly reasonable to be careful about what you share and who you share it with.

As you reconnect with others, you might find you are given a smorgasbord of advice. Eating from a buffet can be a good experience if you choose what you want and don't overeat. Listening to advice can be a similar experience. It is important to remind yourself that it is ultimately your choice as to what counsel you take on board and that you don't want to take on board too much. It is up to you what steps you take and when you take them. Your healing journey is about what is best for you. It isn't about pleasing others.

If you have suffered loss in your life, ask yourself, "Has my loss stopped me from living my story? Has it disconnected me from the world that surrounds me?" If the answer is yes, what do you think you need to do?

In addition to personal loss, often we can find ourselves in a place where someone we care about a great deal has suffered loss and is in a state of grief. In supporting someone in the grieving process, there are a number of ways you can help, but it is important to be aware of the savior complex outlined in the previous chapter and how to appropriately support someone in crisis. Support someone in grief in these ways:

- Be a good listener.
- Respect the person's way of grieving.
- Accept mood swings.
- Avoid giving advice.
- Refrain from trying to explain the loss.
- Help out with practical tasks.
- Stay in touch.
- Be available.

In traditional Aboriginal society, the entire community was involved in the grieving and healing process. This included specific ceremonies, songs, and dances that would be carried out, sometimes for long periods of time.

In contemporary Aboriginal society, there has been significant intergenerational loss, including loss of culture, loss of traditional life, loss of language, loss of land, loss of children, loss of Lore, loss of identity, loss of independence, loss of purpose, loss of learning systems, and loss of knowledge. Many Aboriginal communities are in a continuous state of pain and suffering as a result.

The Aboriginal experience of loss is also a worldwide experience, because when you think about what the world has lost, many places have lost their connection to their Country and their language. This might be an unconscious loss, where people are unaware of their loss. But it still has an impact on their lives today. Their lost connection to Country means their relationships with their place and all things in their place is gone. My view on healing for our communities is firstly to connect back to Country. So we all must first start on a journey to find that connection. We do that by first looking at who we are and where we come from. Who are our ancestors and what was their responsibility to place and all things in their place? What is our responsibility? The deeper we go into this, the more we realize that our place is what we should be looking after.

Because at the moment we are living on the land like fleas on a dog's back. We are parasites. We are taking and not giving.

We need to become part of the land again, and the only way to do this is through the ancient spiritual connection our ancestors had all over the world. Through slowly reconnecting with our story, taking one step at a time, looking and listening to people who can guide us, and learning, we might reach that full connection and understanding once again. This is a time for renewal. This starts at a community level.

Many people in communities come up and say to me, "Our community used to be a good place once." So if we remember the story of our community when it was a good place, as a community, all we have to do is come together and remember that story, share that story, and bring that story back. Just like individuals can be in depression, communities can be in depression. Most individuals with depression can remember when they were in a good place and most of them can remember when that good place was taken from them. Communities are the same.

Coming together and sharing the stories of when our community was a good place will allow us to bring that good place back. Without remembering the past, an individual or a community can never heal.

Each day provides us with literally hundreds of opportunities to enjoy the moment and feel alive. Connecting with your senses, finding beauty in everyday things, laughing at silliness, not worrying about what others think, and doing something you enjoy just for the sake of it are ways to live each day with purpose and good intent rather than in mindless endurance. It is up to you to make this a priority.

Accepting our past and learning from it will give us valuable insights into how we harvest the now. To do this, we also need to acknowledge our scars and address them if they are preventing us from walking our footsteps. We can only walk our footsteps in the present moment. Where we are heading is an unknown. We can plan a future but we don't really know what is up ahead . . . so there is no point fixating on it.

Loss is an agonizing experience: it occurred in the past, is felt in the present, and awaits us in the future. It is an inevitable cyclone we must all face at points in our life. Our personal healing journey and those of communities, countries, and the planet are an interwoven web that we must reflect on and commit to.

By understanding the teachings of the Lore and connecting to the Dreaming Path, we are able to better reflect on, understand, and appreciate our own story and, in so doing, implement change that will improve our personal well-being and our ability to generate well-being in our communities.

Message 19

Your past is an important path to your present. Acknowledge, accept, and learn from your past and address those things that are preventing you from finding contentment in the now.

Message 20

Too much focus on the future distracts you from the magic of the present.

Message 21

Embrace change.

Message 22

Laugh often.

Message 23

When loss occurs, allow yourself to grieve and heal.

Chapter 7

Contentment

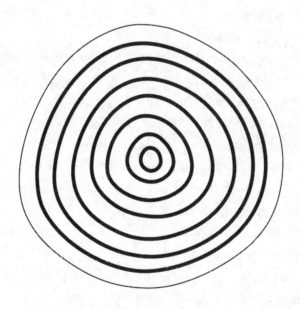

Weda was a clever man, a man of great magic. But he and his wife, Bullen Bullen, were never happy with what they had. Each day, they would wake up early before anyone else was awake and go to gather pretty things to put around their ngurra, their camp.

Of all the many things they liked, they liked things that glittered and sparkled most of all. When no one else in the tribe was watching or when the people had left their camps, they would steal pretty things.

The men would come back to their place and say, "Where is my ceremonial belt?"

The women would come back to their place and say, "Where is my special necklace?"

When the people realized that it was Weda and Bullen Bullen who had stolen their things, they decided to punish them both. The tribe gathered their coolamon dishes and filled them with red-hot coals.

"If Weda and Bullen Bullen want shiny things, they can have these red-hot coals," they said.

The people arrived at Weda's camp and said to the two, "Come outside, we have shiny gifts for you."

As the two stepped outside, they saw many coolamons and became very excited when they saw that inside them were things that sparkled and glowed like the sun.

The tribe threw the coals in the air and they rained down on Weda and Bullen Bullen, who were dancing with joy until they realized it was fire. To avoid being killed, they used their magic to turn themselves into bowerbirds and they flew away.

To this day, Weda the bowerbird builds a bower of grass and gathers shiny things and steals pretty things to put around his camp. But he is still not content.

Bullen Bullen is not content either. She comes and looks at what he has gathered and always says, "That is not pretty enough. I think I will look for a new husband and a new camp." So Weda still gathers pretty things, thinking it will bring contentment to him and Bullen Bullen—thinking that will make them both happy.

Most of us tend to focus more on the negative as we try to make sense of the world. Don't be hard on yourself for doing this: it is part of our brain's way of processing information and warning us of potential threats. Psychologists refer to this as "negative bias." This way of thinking and behaving means that we tend to:

- remember unfavorable experiences more than positive ones,
- recall insults better than praise,
- react more strongly to negative stimuli than to positive stimuli,
- think about negative things more than positive things, and
- respond more strongly to negative events than to equally positive ones.

If our brain is wired so strongly to focus on the negative, is it any wonder we find it so hard to feel contented?

Most people would describe feeling contented as being satisfied or happy with their life, and in many instances people are. But are we as contented as we ought to be or can be?

In traditional Aboriginal society, achieving a state of contentment was a given. The integration of spirituality and the Lore into a child's upbringing meant that they transitioned into adult life with all they needed to live a good story.

My Dreaming is about my life and what I do with it. It can't exist without the connection to the Dreaming of my ancestors through the Dreaming Path.

My Dreaming should show my connection to the past through my connection to the stories of my place and those who have come before me. My Dreaming should not take away from what they left me to care for. I must honor their footprints.

My Dreaming should benefit all things rather than take away from all things. So part of my Dreaming is to pass on the knowledge about the land and all things that I have been taught. Because knowledge is powerful only when shared. And if I believe I have something good, I should give it away so others will benefit from it.

Your Dreaming is about your life and what you do with it. What do you want to leave behind? Do you want to leave behind nothing? Do you want to leave behind destruction? Or do you want to leave behind something positive, something real and something good for the next generation?

Think about your life as a tree, a Dreaming Tree. The first thing you must do is put down strong roots. From there you need a strong trunk and then thick branches full of leaves and fruit that can be shared with the next generation.

The roots gather nutrients from their surrounds to grow. Many little things share in the roots, taking from the roots but never killing the roots. Many creatures live in the trunk, using it for food and shelter. Many creatures live in the branches. Together they are all sharing your Dreaming and you are sharing theirs. You are not alone. You are one with all that is around you and with you. You are special.

Our Dreaming, what we do with our life, how we walk our footsteps, and how we live our story, is built from our sense of purpose. Without purpose, it is unlikely we can achieve true contentment. Many people struggle to identify their purpose for the reasons already explored in this book. The many different potential futures we have in front of us can make us feel like we are being pulled in myriad directions simultaneously— leading to a feeling of being stretched, exhausted, confused, and anxious.

The importance of living life with purpose has been captured by many others over time, as shown in the quotes below.

Efforts and courage are not enough without purpose and direction.
—JOHN F. KENNEDY

The soul which has no fixed purpose in life is lost; to be everywhere is to be nowhere.
—MICHEL DE MONTAIGNE

The best way to lengthen out our days is to walk steadily and with a purpose.

—CHARLES DICKENS

True happiness is not attained through self-gratification, but through fidelity to a worthy purpose.

—HELEN KELLER

The man without a purpose is like a ship without a rudder.

—THOMAS CARLYLE

The heart of human excellence often begins to beat when you discover a pursuit that absorbs you, frees you, challenges you, or gives you a sense of meaning, joy, or passion.

—TERRY ORLICK

The mystery of human existence lies not in just staying alive, but in finding something to live for.

—FYODOR DOSTOYEVSKY

Musicians must make music, artists must paint, poets must write if they are ultimately to be at peace with themselves. What humans can be they must be.

—ABRAHAM MASLOW

These quotes provide clues to how we can identify our purpose. They suggest our purpose is built around what:

- absorbs us,
- gives us a sense of joy,
- we are passionate about,
- gives a sense of freedom when we think about it or do it,

- gives us something to live for,
- enables us to be at peace with ourselves, and
- captures our sense of what we must be.

Our purpose enables us to wake up and look forward to the day ahead.

We are all different, so how each of us delineates our life purpose can differ as well. It doesn't really matter whether we write it as a statement, draw it as a picture, or see it as an overarching bubble of words. What is important is that we have one that feels right, that we believe in, and that inspires us each day.

From an Aboriginal perspective, our purpose and therefore our platform for contentment is about the journey rather than the destination. Some people might roll their eyes and say this sounds like a New Age cliché. To do this is dismissive and foolish. Wisdom is wisdom, regardless of how cheesy it might sound.

If you think about life, the ultimate destination point that awaits us in physical form is death. If you knew you had only forty-eight hours to live, would your focus be on getting to the end as quickly as possible or would you try to slow time down so you could savor every second as best you could? Would you focus on the destination (death) or the journey (the precious moment of now)?

For our Old People, the journey—upholding the Lore each moment in time, including celebrating the now—was what life was about. Death was therefore not something to be feared; regardless of when the time came, a good story had been lived (there was no last-minute rush to make amends, seek atonement, or try to leave a lasting legacy).

For Aboriginal people, purpose and contentment was achieved by ensuring each day that they:

- cared for Country,
- respected all things,
- maintained rich relationships with people and place,
- shared all they had,
- nurtured connectedness and unity,
- loved all things and converted this into action,
- lived with gratitude,
- were humble in all actions,
- were inspired in all actions,
- lived in the present,
- honored the past,
- upheld the Lore, and
- fulfilled their responsibilities.

These actions fit within an Aboriginal worldview that is somewhat different to the Western worldview, as show in the table on the next page. We acknowledge that this table is generic in nature and that we are all individuals with unique and diverse views and values. The information, however, provides a useful conceptual platform for us to reflect on in terms of what drives our behavior.

Neither worldview is wrong or right; they are just different. Most of us live in the right-hand-column world, but there are attributes of the left-hand-column world that many of us might think can contribute to improved individual, community, national, and global well-being. The obvious question is "How can we bring the two columns together?"

Aboriginal Worldview	Western Worldview
Spiritual beliefs embedded in all aspects of life	Spirituality may or may not be important
Story, song, dance, and art are the platform of learning	Science and evidence-based knowledge form the platform of learning
Society is interrelated– connectivity to all things is central to being	Society is sectionalized– connectivity is based on need
Flow-ers: adept at reading their environment and flowing with it	Achievers: doing is important; adept at changing their environment to service need
Identity comes from connections and culture (Lore, language, Country, family, ceremony)	Identity comes from jobs and material possessions
Time is nonsequential and observed through nature; lifestyle flows with time	Time is ordered and monitored through gadgetry; lifestyle fights with time
Authority based on cultural knowledge and use of that knowledge to help others	Authority based on roles assigned through systems
Contentment achieved through meaningful relationships and upholding of the Lore	Contentment achieved through achieving goals

Responsibilities and obligations are an important part of walking our footsteps and living our Dreaming. How we view the world will dictate what we feel responsible for and obliged to do.

Aboriginal spirituality cannot be separated from nature, cannot be separated from everyday actions, cannot be separated from the past, cannot be separated from the present, and cannot be separated from the future. It is entwined in all aspects of our life, including our purpose.

Aboriginal spirituality is about the connectedness of all things and the obligations all things have to each other. It isn't a specific thing. It is all things. It is the law of obligation and responsibility to all things.

In the Aboriginal world, you have a story, song, and dance and they are all connected with each other. These stories tell us our obligations. Our obligations to rocks, trees, fish, birds, and animals. Our obligations to everything, including each other.

But the traditional Aboriginal world wasn't only about our obligations to what we have down here on earth; it was also about our obligations to all the things in the sky as well. So when you look up into the sky in the nighttime and you see stars, there are stories about the stars. When you see the moon, there is a story about the moon, and when you see the sun, there are stories about the sun. So everything we could see or touch had a story, a song, a dance—and obligations.

In traditional Aboriginal times, responsibility was embedded in all aspects of daily life. These responsibilities could include upholding the Lore (caring for my place and all things in my place), sharing knowledge, participating in ceremony, building shelter, gathering and preparing food, and a host of other activities.

We all have responsibilities—such as being the best person we can be, caring for our family, carrying out work duties, continually growing our knowledge base, and maintaining friendships—but how often do we sit down and think about them?

Exercise: Responsibilities

On a blank sheet of paper, write down all of your personal responsibilities. If it helps, you might think about your responsibilities in these and other key areas.

- You
- Family
- Employment
- Education
- Financial security
- Social connection
- Other

Now think about responsibility and obligation from an Aboriginal perspective; that is, "caring for your place and all things in your place." This brings into play key areas such as environmental, community, and global responsibilities.

Are there any responsibilities you need to add to your list? This might include things you need to do for better self-care.

Once you have completed your list, review it in the context of a reality check. Are your responsibilities reasonable and manageable? If the answer is no, you might have an insight into why you might feel overwhelmed at times.

Go back through the responsibilities and categorize them as either C (critical for me to carry out), NE (not essential for me to do but important), and U (unimportant in the scheme of things). In doing this, challenge yourself as to whether the responsibilities reflect your truth or whether they reflect other people's expectations.

What do you need to do to ensure your responsibilities can be met in a way that supports emotional and spiritual balance and well-being? Do you need to delete, share, delegate, or seek support for any of them?

Now finalize your list of responsibilities and create a plan of how you can fulfill them in a way that adds to your well-being rather than undermines it.

Given we are born into this world with a life purpose, it follows that fulfilling our responsibilities should be a rewarding experience (if purpose and responsibilities are in alignment).

From an Aboriginal spiritual perspective, although there will be times when we are challenged (part of our learning), carrying out our responsibilities should add to our feeling of well-being each day. Carrying out our responsibilities should not undermine our well-being with out-of-control busyness and stress.

If we are living a good story, our life will be in balance. If it becomes out of balance, our ability to feel peace or contentment is severely compromised. We can be leached of color and our world becomes gray.

To avoid this, it is important that we take ownership of our well-being rather than be a victim of what surrounds us.

We need to learn to look out for ourselves and take care of ourselves.

Exercise: Self-Care

Listed below are a number of elements relating to good self-care. Rate yourself out of five for each element. Five means you are a master, and one means you aren't very good at that element at this point in time.

General

- I engage in activities and practices that give me energy, lower my stress, and contribute to my well-being.
- I monitor how I am traveling mentally, physically, and spiritually.
- I am very committed to my health and well-being.
- I identify and act on my learning needs.
- I regularly connect with a mentor.
- I celebrate special occasions.
- I express my needs and seek help where appropriate.

Psychological

- When I find myself rushing, I am able to slow myself down.
- When I find myself feeling like life is a chore, I can change my self-talk to reflect gratitude.
- I embrace change.
- I feel empowered.
- I am good at making decisions.
- I make time for recreation/relaxation/a hobby.
- I regularly connect with positive family members and friends.

Physical

- I have a good sleep routine.
- I maintain a healthy diet.
- I exercise each day.

Spiritual

- I regularly meditate/empty my mind.
- I regularly walk in the bush.

- I regularly engage in a religious or spiritual service/practice/ceremony.

Work
- I have good work-life balance.
- I set boundaries.
- I make sure I have regular self-care breaks during the day.
- I ensure that I don't overextend myself on a regular basis.
- I start my day by identifying my priorities.
- I turn off my work phone and don't look at my email after work.
- When I finish work for the day, I can detach from it.

What are you good at?

What are the priority areas you need to work on? What do you need to do?

How will you ensure you do what you need to do?

Creating a healthy mind, body, and spirit requires focus and commitment. It also requires flexibility. In traditional Aboriginal life, the Lore provided structure and stability—but in a way that promoted flexibility so the individual and tribe could feel, respond to, and live in harmony with the ebbs, flows, and heartbeat of the land.

To get things done in our lives, we need a degree of structure, continuity, and consistency. It is important, however, that we don't become robots or build lives that are totally programmed and inflexible. We need to flow like water—to reach our destination by calmly winding and meandering in synchronicity with what is around us. By doing this, we experience a plethora of topographies, learning with each twist and turn about many things we did not know even existed.

Increasing your ability to meander and flow might include these strategies:

- Take an extra thirty minutes away from the workplace to enjoy someone's company or a walk in the park.
- Enjoy a piece of chocolate, even when you are focused on your physical health and fitness.
- Stop midway through a jog to smell a rose.
- Take time out from washing the dishes to watch a sunset.
- Turn off social media and call someone to tell them you are thinking about them.
- Go for a drive with no idea where you are heading.
- Try a new food.
- Connect with the arts.
- Take a morning bath.
- Watch clouds.
- Do something spontaneous that is outside your comfort zone.
- Talk to a stranger.

These kinds of opportunities abound every day; it is a matter of having the intent, courage, belief, faith, and self-permission to harvest them.

In order to develop this mindset, it helps if your basic needs are met, of course. Lack of access to basic needs—such as housing, income, work, social interaction, education, transportation, good health, and personal safety—is a reality for many people.

Those of us who do not face these hardships have an obligation to think about how to make the world a more equitable place for all people. From an Aboriginal spiritual perspective, living a good story means no one is left behind.

Acknowledging our good fortune, appreciating how lucky we are, and feeling special every day are great things to do. Even if we achieve this state of being, however, we won't feel happy every moment of every day. A far better expectation is to have the ability to ride the peaks and troughs of life as they invariably arrive.

Although it is important to take action when we are able to, the reality is there will be times when things happen that are beyond our control. This is where accepting the situation and not "awfulizing" about what has happened will help you move through the storm and find the calm that awaits on the other side.

Through accepting what is happening in your life (good and bad), not pressuring yourself to feel abundantly joyful at all times, and harvesting the magic in every day, you have a sound base from which you can work toward your life purpose with belief in your ability to respond to any unforeseen challenges in an appropriate and confident way.

Now you have insights into the importance of purpose, responsibilities, self-care, and flexibility in achieving contentment in your life, you are ready to start to contemplate life goals. These are goals that capture our ambitions by describing what we would like to achieve in our life. They identify aims and results we are willing to commit effort to. We all have them. Usually, they are unwritten and in the back of our minds. This lack of visibility means they can be easily or conveniently forgotten.

Your Dreaming is a journey that flows without rush and with reverence for the present moment. At the same time, it is important that your Dreaming is consistent and has direction. Goals can help you with your direction and ensure you don't lose sight of what is important to you.

When the journey of your life approaches its autumn, imagine being able to look back and feel good about where you have been, what you have learned, and what you have done. Imagine being able to say to yourself that you have lived the best story possible, walked your footsteps and embraced your unique palette of colors at all times. Setting goals will point you in that direction.

Some people believe that fulfilling your destiny isn't about aiming for anything in particular. They argue our destiny is already set—that contentment is about freeing our spirit and trusting where the journey takes us. I must say I have one foot in that camp of thought. At the same time, it is possible to set broad goals in a way that supports this approach to life.

Our life's journey is a bit like traveling down a beautiful river in a canoe. There will be times when it is OK to lay the paddle gently down and let the canoe drift along with the current so we can take in everything around us. Sometimes, however, the current might take us to a still part of the river and, when the time is right, we will need to pick up the paddle so we can start moving again. As we resume our journey along the river, we might come across some rapids. Our paddle may be necessary once again—to ensure we don't capsize and place ourselves at risk.

Taking ownership of your life means there will be times when you have to be active rather than passive. You might need to undertake some studies, submit a job application, seek help, say no to a request, or make changes in your life.

The challenge is to know when to paddle and when to float. Our Old People teach us that our intuition will guide us if we listen to it and trust it.

Setting a small number of life goals can be challenging, particularly if you are feeling lost. If you see this as an opportunity to reflect, contemplate, and explore, rather than something you have to get right the first time, you might find the process a liberating one. Your goals are to you . . . from you . . . about you . . . and you can change them whenever you feel the need.

Exercise: Life Goals

On a blank piece of paper write down the following question: *When I am eighty-five years old and I look back on my life, how would I like people to describe my story?*

Once you have written this down, read the words again and let them gently soak into your conscious mind with no particular focus or intent.

Close your eyes and for a minute or two let different pictures, words, and thoughts flow without judgment or boundary. Allow yourself to dream.

When you are ready, write down words that capture the essence of how you want your story to read.

Repeat the process above for the question: *What is important to me and what excites me?*

Repeat the process above for the question: *If I knew I could not fail, what would I like to achieve?*

Look at the answers you have written down to the three questions and identify the themes that are most important to you. Narrow down your list to five themes and convert them into goals.

An example of a goal is as follows: *I will live a life of gratitude that will include recognizing the blessings I have every day.*

Now that you have identified some goals, it is time to identify what actions you need to take to achieve them. After you have done this, for each goal, you can reflect on whether you are on track, heading the wrong way, or need to start from scratch.

Regardless of where you are with each of them, remind yourself how good it is to have some direction in your life. You can now commit to changes you need to make in your life knowing they align with your life purpose and goals that are long-term, meaningful, personal, powerful, and based on your truth.

This knowledge will give you renewed energy, motivation, and enthusiasm to charge into each day with an enhanced drive to deal with whatever challenges you might face, because you have a cause you believe in—you. As you take your first steps, think about how good it is to leave clear, distinct, purposeful footprints in the sand and allow the anticipation and excitement to inspire you.

In doing this, it is important to understand that taking ownership of your life, your footsteps, your decisions, and your actions each moment of each day can be a double-edged sword. It means you have to also take ownership of the consequences of your decisions and actions. It is easy to blame others when things go wrong (and, to be fair, sometimes things do go wrong because of others), but our reactions when things don't go according to plan are what define us and they lay the foundation for our peace of mind and contentment.

If we accept what is happening around us with objectivity, patience, and a positive attitude (What can I learn from this? . . . This storm will pass . . . What are my next steps?), then we will hold on to our power and find owning the consequences of our decisions is just as freeing as owning the decisions themselves. This freedom will reduce fear to the point you might even become fearless. If you are fearless, you will find peace of mind easier to access.

Your story—your Dreaming—is a journey, remember. For more than 60,000 years, Aboriginal people have continually journeyed through Country in order to harvest its bounty, conduct ceremony, and ensure sustainability of the flora and fauna living on it. In Aboriginal spirituality, our life is a journey and when it is finished in this physical form, we journey back to the stars to rest before starting on another journey.

Given our life is a journey and subject to continuous change internally (the way we think) and externally (what is happening around us), it is important and healthy to regularly review our life goals and our progress toward them so we don't drift off course.

If we don't notice the drift, we might feel agitated and unsettled without knowing why and continue with life as if nothing is wrong. If we don't address how we are feeling, our dissatisfaction might grow, leading to Band-Aid behaviors, including:

- blaming others
- looking for a new job
- buying a new car
- getting a divorce or having an affair

- falling into a habit of complaining to others
- working harder and longer
- self-medicating
- putting others' needs and interests before our own

Eventually, we open ourselves up to the potential for a personal crisis. A midlife crisis is often described as a transition of identity and self-confidence that can occur in middle-aged individuals, typically forty-five to fifty-five years old. It is usually viewed as a psychological crisis triggered by an individual contemplating their mortality, achievements (or lack of achievements), and overall contentment with life as it is. From an Aboriginal perspective, this kind of crisis is symptomatic of a person who has realized they are not living a good story. The fact that the person is in crisis is therefore of no great surprise.

There are a number of other triggers that can create a crisis such that an individual reconsiders their life journey. Examples of these triggers include:

- the death of a family member
- a health scare (either for us or someone we love)
- unemployment
- children leaving home
- marital separation
- menopause

One of my favorite sayings is "Don't waste a good crisis." When one arises, contemplating your hopes and dreams, your life purpose, and whether you are happy with your current trajectory is a healthy and productive thing to do. From this reflection, you might identify new things you want to do with your life and turn the negative situation into a positive one. This doesn't take away from the grief of the initial trigger, of course, but if you can benefit from what is happening, it makes sense to do so.

But why wait for a crisis to generate the reflection process? It is never too early or too late to assess our journey and whether we think we are on track. When carrying out this assessment, try to do so in an objective, unbiased, nonattached way. If you review your life so far with judgment and negativity, it will be hard for you to identify the silver lining in the clouds of the past. It will be difficult to address those things that are not resolved, so you can heal, learn, grow, and go forward.

When we allow ourselves to be seduced by negativity, our inner dialogues can inundate us with a variety of distortions, including all-or-nothing thinking; labeling; overgeneralizing; assuming; ruminating; unfavorable comparing; catastrophizing; personalizing; blaming; minimizing the good; magnifying the bad; and shoulds, oughts, and musts.

It isn't essential to understand these various distortions. They are provided just to help you appreciate how significantly unhelpful our brain can be to our well-being. Given our mental chatter is up to 70 percent negative, it is useful to understand how to turn the volume down.

Exercise: Quieting the Mind

Listed below are a number of ways you can begin working on quieting the negative talk of your mind (sometimes described as "monkey mind" chatter). Take as much time as you need to think about each of the items listed and how they might relate to you. After you have done this, choose one item only and convert it into a written action that you will carry out for at least two weeks.

After two weeks have elapsed, review your progress and, if appropriate, choose another item and do the same thing.

Continue working through the list (for the rest of your life if need be).

- Watch out for the distorted stories your mind tries to tell you and acknowledge to yourself they have no place in your life.
- Explore therapeutic support with a professional.
- Meditate.
- Watch your mental chatter without judgment.
- Push back when you find yourself applying negative self-labels.
- Walk Country.
- Exercise.
- Visualize your inner voice as something that looks comical or ridiculous.
- Write down what your inner voice is saying and assess whether what it is saying is helpful. If it isn't, reframe the words. For example, "The project failed because of me" might become "This is the first time any of us have attempted this. Next time all of us will know how to do this, and I will feel more confident."
- Read a book.
- Don't assume you know what another person is thinking about you.
- Remind yourself you have had negative thoughts in the past and have not only survived them but have had positive feelings and experiences since.

- Listen to music you love and maybe even sing along.
- Distance yourself from the thought, then imagine one of your friends is thinking this way about themself. Think about what you would say to them.
- Remind yourself your thoughts don't rule you. You can listen to what your inner voice is saying but you don't have to agree with it.
- Don't compare yourself with other people.

Given we grow up in a world of continuous and often fierce competition, it can be very easy to slip into the habit of comparing ourselves with others. In doing this we fail to appreciate how unique each of us is, how we each radiate an individual fingerprint of dynamic color, and how we each have a distinct and amazing Dreaming to walk.

Comparing ourselves to others undermines our ability to achieve contentment.

An important part of our culture is corroboree. This is when we come together and dance. There was a big corroboree many years ago where we had more than a hundred dancers and an audience of more than a thousand people. As the dancers were getting ready, I noticed one man sitting down looking very nervous. It was the first time he was going to dance at a public corroboree.

I went over to him and asked him how he was. "I am so nervous, I think I am going to be sick," he said. I laughed and asked him why he was so nervous. "Because there are going to be two thousand eyes watching me and I can't dance as well as the others," he replied.

I asked him, "Who do you think you are dancing for?"

He pointed to the crowd and said, "All those people, of course. I just told you that."

I shook my head and pointed to the trees. "What do you see?" I said to him.

"I see the trees moving with the wind," he said.

"And why is there such a big wind that wasn't there earlier?" I asked.

He replied, "Because of all the Old Spirits coming in to watch us."

"That is all you need to think about when you dance tonight," I told him. "When you dance, you dance for the Old Spirits. You don't dance for the audience. It is good that they are here, but that is not why we do what we do. So when you go out there, you connect with those Old Spirits and dance for them. Don't go worrying about the other dancers and how they dance and how good they are. If you connect with those Old Ones, the way you move will be perfect."

That man was Paul Callaghan, the author of this book. It was his fortieth birthday and he told me later what he learned that night was the best birthday present. He learned to believe in himself, he learned to believe in his actions, and he learned not to compare himself with others.

The negative bias of our brain means we are always scanning what is around us to identify potential danger. Being intimidated by others can occur as a result. By knowing this and challenging our self-talk, we can reshape our negativity and:

- start recognizing our successes,
- stop comparing ourselves to other people,
- value ourselves as we are, and
- do what we believe is right without worrying about what others might say or think.

By challenging our thoughts, we will have increased clarity and confidence in our footsteps and be better equipped to let go of the negative mind chatter that can impede optimism and positivity.

Exercise: What Does Contentment Mean to Me?

Listed below are a number of quotes relating to contentment. Review each of them and, on a blank piece of paper, write down words that resonate with you.

Comparison makes finding contentment a million times harder.

Contentment is not the fulfillment of what you want but the realization of how much you already have.

Realize that true happiness lies within you. Waste no time and effort searching for something only to realize you had it with you the whole time.

If one's life is simple, contentment has to come. Simplicity is extremely important for happiness. Having few desires, feeling satisfied with what you have, is very vital: satisfaction with just enough food, clothing, and shelter to protect yourself from the elements. And finally, there is an intense delight in

*abandoning faulty states of mind and in cultivating healthy ones
in meditation.*

—DALAI LAMA

Contentment is natural wealth; luxury is artificial poverty.

—SOCRATES

*Just become totally content and happy from within. Then you
will get all that you want.*

—SRI SRI RAVI SHANKAR

Patience is the key to contentment.

—THE PROPHET MUHAMMAD

*Life is about balance. Be kind, but don't let people abuse you.
Trust, but don't be deceived. Be content, but never stop improving
yourself.*

—UNKNOWN

Now write a sentence or paragraph that reflects what contentment
means to you.

By understanding our brain's negative biases, identifying our
purpose, bringing together the Aboriginal and Western worldviews, defining our responsibilities, making self-care a priority, being flexible, setting life goals, knowing how to quiet our mind, and
creating our own definition of contentment, we are able to find a
place of peace within, regardless of what storms might arrive.

Although contentment isn't about being happy all the time, being happy is still a good thing to embrace. There are many things we can do:

- Set realistic expectations.
- Smile.
- Be grateful.
- Walk Country.
- Let go of worry and grudges.
- Practice self-care.
- Give back.
- Be flexible and experiment.
- Take your time.
- Exercise, eat well, and get plenty of sleep.
- Have a purpose.
- Give compliments.
- Face things that are troubling you.
- Visit friends.
- Plan a trip.
- Reflect, learn, and grow.
- Be present.
- Meditate.
- Turn the phone off.

If you think about traditional Aboriginal people and their approach to life, you will find that they practiced all the good habits listed above (with the exception of the phone, of course).

No one person, group, book, video, program, or organization has the entire solution to the challenges you will face in living the best story possible. You will certainly benefit from the wisdom and support of others, but ultimately it is up to you to decide what works for you. So don't be afraid to be the author of your story, to own your future and trust your judgment.

The river never stays the same; it is forever changing, as are the Mother and all her children. Remember you are one of her children: loved, cared for, but given autonomy and choice in what you want to do with your life.

We are born into this world to live a good story and follow our Dreaming. In today's world, there are many obstacles we need to navigate in order to do this. With understanding, patience, and determination we can take our next steps forward knowing that by focusing on the journey, we bring contentment within our grasp.

Message 24

Your Dreaming is about your life and what you do with it. Part of your Dreaming is to connect to the Dreaming Path.

Message 25

View the world from beyond the Western perspective. By learning from other cultures, you will live a more fulfilling story and help create a better world.

Message 26

To care for others, we need to first care for ourselves.

Message 27

We need to flow like water. We reach our destination by calmly accepting the twists and turns ahead of us and adjusting our course as we see fit.

Message 28

Living a good story means no one gets left behind.

Message 29

Don't give your power away to the chatter of your mind.

Chapter 8

Leading

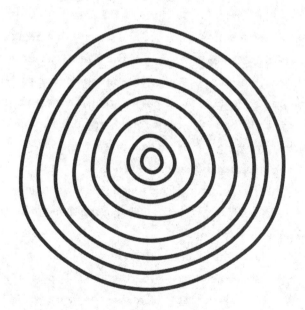

It was a time of deep sadness. All of the animals did their best to support each other after Grandfather Eagle had passed to the spirit world, but it felt like a big hole had been left that couldn't be filled.

Animals came from far and wide to pay their respects to Grandfather Eagle. He had much wisdom and had used his knowledge to help many over the years. "Farewell, my brother," Grandfather Owl said. "You have lived a very good story."

After Sorry Business finished and Grandfather Eagle's spirit was on its way, a meeting of the clan was called and the animals gathered. They had to choose someone to replace Grandfather Eagle at the Great Meeting, the meeting where clans from far and wide came together to discuss important things. A meeting was being held that afternoon.

"Who shall lead us?" said Bandicoot.

"Our Elders, of course," his friend Wallaby said, looking over to the Elders, who were sitting in the shade of a big gum tree, quietly watching.

"Yes, I know the Elders guide us on all things, but who will sit in the Great Meeting and represent us?" Bandicoot asked.

"Well, if we sit and listen, I am sure the Elders will tell us," Wallaby replied.

There was quiet for a while as everybody waited for the Elders to speak.

"Why should it be an Elder?" Frilled-Neck Lizard said, breaking the silence in a very bossy voice. "I'm a bit sick and tired of the Old People giving me orders. It's about time a young person like me had a say. It's about time we had new ideas."

The Elders remained silent.

"What makes you think you should be the boss?" Magpie asked Frilled-Neck Lizard.

"Well, for a start, I'm smarter than any of you. And I am also not afraid of anything." After he finished saying this, Frilled-Neck Lizard puffed out his frills and ran in a circle. He looked very fierce and none of the younger animals were game to say a thing. The Elders spoke quietly among themselves as the other animals waited patiently. When they finished speaking, Grandfather Owl hopped over to Frilled-Neck Lizard.

"Off you go, then," Grandfather Owl said. "We are looking forward to hearing you tell us about the meeting later tonight." Frilled-Neck Lizard whooped for joy and ran around all the animals singing, "I'm the boss, I'm the boss, I'm the boss, because I'm the best."

When he finally sat in the circle of the Great Meeting, Frilled-Neck Lizard couldn't wait to have his say. Whenever one of the old bosses spoke, Frilled-Neck Lizard would argue and say they were thinking like dinosaurs and that they needed to move ahead with the times.

"The Lore has done a good job for us for a long time," Frilled-Neck Lizard said to the gathering. "But we need change."

"Give us an example of what we should do differently,"
Grandmother Emu said.

"Well, we can no longer give away things. In our Country,
when the plums grow, we will pick them all, and when
other clans and tribes want some, we will ask them to trade
something like a coolamon or an axe for our food."

"And what happens if they have nothing to trade?"
Grandmother Emu asked.

"Then they can't have any," Frilled-Neck Lizard replied.
"And we will create a special force to stop people from trying
to steal them as well."

The old bosses shook their heads but Frilled-Neck Lizard
wasn't watching.

"And because our fruit is so popular, I think we will clear
some forest and bush and plant seeds. We will have more
fruit than anyone. And if other clans and tribes want to know
how we do it, we won't tell them, but we can take over some
of their Country and grow fruit for them as well. We can
become the biggest tribe of all."

"Enough," said Grandfather Owl as he flew in and joined
the circle. "You have disrespected the Elders and you have
questioned the Lore. You don't want unity and you don't
want to share. You don't respect relationships and you don't
respect Country."

Frilled-Neck Lizard became very angry. "You are wrong.
You are all wrong."

"There is nothing wrong with change, nephew,"
Grandmother Emu said. "But leaders must think about the
consequences of their decisions . . . and they must think

about how their decisions will affect the land and all things on the land long after they are gone."

Grandfather Goanna spoke. "A leader makes a path so it is easier for others to follow. The path you want to create just isn't right, nephew."

Frilled-Neck Lizard was furious. "You are all silly old fools," he said. After he spoke, he ripped a branch off a small tree and threw it to the ground in anger before running off. "I don't need you. I don't need anybody," he said as he scampered over a sand dune, never to be seen again.

As he got older, Frilled-Neck Lizard grew lonely, but if you should come across him, he puffs up his frills to let you know that he is still very angry and he still thinks he should be the boss.

But if you challenge him, he still runs away . . . and the tracks he leaves still aren't the right ones to follow.

Can you imagine what life would be like if we didn't have leaders? Leadership is critical in any society, as leaders drive vision, decisions, actions, and culture.

Leadership is generally considered to be the action of guiding, steering, and influencing a group of people or an organization, or the ability to do this. It ties in closely with the term *governance*, which is about exercising power over how things are done. It goes without saying that good leadership can achieve great things while poor leadership can be disastrous.

Leadership is therefore one of the biggest responsibilities we can have in our lives.

As we go through life, eventually we will be given leadership responsibilities. We become good leaders when we listen, love, and understand people's stories.

You can't become a leader if you don't know anybody's story or if you don't know your own story. The world is full of leaders who have no story, leaders who have no love.

They haven't been taught to look and listen and so they haven't learned the things they need to learn. Yet they're our leaders and so they lead us down the wrong path. They make wrong decisions and they do this over and over again.

A leader is not someone with words but someone with action—action that is attached to real knowledge. The only way you can have real knowledge is by acknowledging your responsibilities (Lore), loving, looking, listening, and learning. I call these the five Ls. By following the five Ls, you have an understanding of who you are, where you are from, and what your role is in the universe. Once you have done this you are ready for the sixth L. You are ready to lead.

If you type the word *leadership* into a search engine, the screen is inundated with descriptors relating to business and organizational environments. The search results indicate that leaders are about maximizing efficiency, attaining organizational goals, and delivering results through others.

If our Old People saw this, they would shake their heads in dismay. They would say where is the love for Country? Where is the love for the animals and the birds, rocks, and trees?

In the Western system, there are a multitude of theories that indicate an effective leader must:

- understand power and influence,
- have excellent people skills,
- be able to identify critical organizational functions,
- promote appropriate values,
- engage everybody in one vision,
- possess high-order analytical skills,
- have a winning personality, and
- be able to communicate effectively.

In traditional times, Aboriginal Elders possessed all the competencies listed above but used their skills in a much different way from that seen in the modern-day boardroom.

The traditional Aboriginal view of leadership is much broader than "delivering results through others." Aboriginal leadership is about "fulfilling my responsibilities, including caring for my place and all things in my place on behalf of my children's children's children's children."

The table below provides insight into some primary differences between Aboriginal leadership and Western leadership.

Western Leadership	Aboriginal Leadership
Focus on staff deficits	Focus on an individual's strengths
Everything is urgent	There is time for whatever needs to be done
Power dominates	Power is shared in a humble, respectful, and loving way
Things measured are more highly valued	Relationships are more highly valued
Worship of the written word	Worship of story and narrative

Western Leadership	Aboriginal Leadership
Only one right way	Many right ways
Success is measured by achieving KPIs (usually related to internal measurables, including revenue, profit, and asset values)	Success is measured by relationships with other people, the land, the sky, and all living things
Decisions made relate to impacts on business KPIs over the next three years	Decisions made relate to impacts on children's children's children's children

The Elders, who from a Western leadership perspective were the executive leadership team, provided effective leadership for tens of thousands of years. The governance system our people used ensured that authority and power weren't abused.

The question you might ask is "Does the Aboriginal way of leading have any application in the contemporary world of global markets, supply-and-demand-driven services, consumerism, and cash flow?"

The answer is yes, particularly when you consider the emergence of the concept of corporate citizenship and the pressure on organizations to be good corporate citizens. The term itself was coined in the 1970s but is becoming increasingly important as both individual and institutional investors seek out companies that are socially responsible. Corporate citizenship is about a company's responsibility to manage not only financial performance but also produce higher standards of living and better quality of life for the communities that surround them, particularly with regards to environmental and social issues.

More and more organizations are demonstrating good corporate social responsibility. In many ways, the activities being carried out by these organizations reflect Aboriginal ways of thinking and acting:

- reducing carbon footprints (caring for the Mother)
- donating to charitable organizations (sharing)
- volunteering (connectivity, relationships, community well-being)
- supporting the environment (caring for Country)
- targeted social causes, such as mental health, addressing disadvantage, climate action, and Indigenous well-being (caring for our place and all things in our place)

It is pleasing to see that forward-thinking corporations have begun to embrace a wider view of what leadership responsibility encompasses. By focusing on social, environmental, cultural, ethical, and equity issues in addition to their financial and economic health, organizations will start becoming givers to, rather than takers from, the societal well-being balance sheet.

This broadening of strategic and operational scope enhances the interconnectivity and alignment between organizational, community, and environmental sustainability and creates a win-win-win. This is important, given that if organizations or communities or the environment are unwell, we are all unwell.

Leadership that embraces a holistic view of relationships (including connections that enhance community and environmental well-being) is therefore critical.

In traditional times, although Aboriginal people endured hardship every now and then, they did so together. No one was disadvantaged when compared to others. In contemporary society, this is not the case. There are some people who, for a variety of reasons, are subject to inequality.

A society committed to well-being for all understands this reality and is committed to addressing it. Community leaders, government leaders, and nongovernment leaders all have important roles to play in addressing disadvantage and creating equity.

There is an abundance of knowledge in our world, including all the knowledge needed to create a better world for all. What is missing is the collective will to transform knowledge into wisdom into leadership action. In addition to addressing basic socioeconomic needs of the many people suffering in this world, we also need our leaders to stand together globally as a matter of human survival—as shown by the number of crises the world is facing at this moment in time, including:

- collaborating to plan for and contain global pandemics,
- renewed arms race and potential for the growth of nuclear weapons,
- international tensions and conflicts,
- the climate crisis,
- energy,
- food and hunger,
- population,
- natural resources,
- global debt and potential recession, and
- cyber-enabled disinformation campaigns.

The number, scale, and profound nature of these crises is a major cause of concern and a strong argument for the need for our leaders to embrace a broader view of leadership—one that reflects the Dreaming Path's mandate: to care for our place and all things in our place above all else. This doesn't discount the many complex drivers of world economies and how nations function, but they need to be framed by a vision and unity of purpose that incorporates a much broader spectrum of well-being.

So look at a world leader. If that world leader doesn't know their Country from its creation and doesn't know its natural order, how can they understand and love the land? How can they lead people if they don't know what all the people want or what all the people need?

If a leader's life revolves around money, prestige, or power, rather than Lore, how can they care and make decisions for the environment and for the majority of the people? In the first L, Lore, our basic need is food, water, and shelter. All this is given to us if we connect to Country and respect all other creatures, along with the living landscape. In the Aboriginal world, rocks are born, rocks have babies, and rocks die—all things have spirit. Yet, in many places, leaders allow the rocks to be mined, smashed, and killed without any regard to spirit. Until one fully understands the depth of the Lore, the obligations and responsibilities that arise and the consequences of not following the Lore, how can one be a leader of a country?

A leader loves. Through understanding their Country in a truly spiritual way, they will learn to love all things in Country, in nature, and realize all things have a right to be.

A leader should take the time to look and listen to all of their people. They need to hear what is important to their people.

They should look at the land and the environment and realize how important it is for them and their people's survival. They need to listen to what the trees and the rocks and the rivers and all things are trying to tell them.

Because without these things, no one will exist. Humanity should not exalt itself above nature.

All leaders have a responsibility to provide all people (regardless of race, color, nation of origin, gender, disability, age, and religion) with the opportunity to live a good story. The Six Ls Model (Lore > Love > Look > Listen > Learn > Lead) provides an overlying framework of principles that can be applied to our leaders so we can have confidence in their ability to make good decisions. It is difficult to have confidence in our leaders if we don't trust what they are saying, trust their motivations, or trust their decisions. When I listen to people around me and look at or listen to the various media platforms (social, television, radio, newspaper) and other sources of public perception, I get the impression that many people don't trust our leaders in government or the corporate sector.

Trust, once broken, can take a long time to be regained. The lack of trust in our leaders is a crisis for all of us. We owe it to ourselves and future generations to demand better.

A review of the history of Australia post-occupation and the effects of successive government policies on Aboriginal people provides an insight into what can happen when leaders do things that they claim are "for" the people rather than "with" the people.

In traditional Aboriginal society, everybody had a sense of worth, everybody had a role to play, and obligations and responsibilities to one another. I see many Aboriginal people today who are lost, not knowing what their purpose is in life because the roles and responsibilities of the generations before them have been taken away.

Most of these men are trying to connect to their culture because they know that, without having that, they will never know where they are going. How can they move forward with no knowledge of who they are?

Governments think that they know what is best for these men, assuming these men want what others have. But before these men can ever know what they want or where they are going, they really have to connect and know the journey that brought them to where they are today.

Before anyone can be educated or employed, they must first be empowered. Empowerment can only be from knowledge, and knowledge comes from the past. Without the knowledge of the past, we can't build on the knowledge of the present, and without the knowledge of the present, we can't foresee our future.

Indigenous peoples throughout the world have had their knowledge forcibly removed from them and another set of knowledge and values imposed on them. By removing the Indigenous story, we have completely disempowered these people. How can a disempowered people move forward? We must allow these people to reconnect with their stories. Only then will they be healed. Only when they are healed can the world be healed.

Throughout my life, I have seen governments waste millions and millions of dollars on housing, health, education, and employment for Aboriginal people. But not one cent was

spent on empowerment for Aboriginal people. They constantly
refuse to listen to or acknowledge our story of loss or address
that loss. While that loss isn't addressed, we will always be
impoverished, poor, and disempowered, and money will continue
to be wasted over and over again.

Governments are elected to lead and provide governance. They have important obligations and responsibilities to each one of us, but are these obligations and responsibilities carried out with knowledge, love, and learning? Are their decisions based on our needs or the needs of those governments to be reelected?

Given our political leaders are elected, there is a critical responsibility for each of us of voting age to:

- understand the purpose of government;
- respect the importance of having the right to vote;
- take the voting process seriously, including studying what candidates are offering;
- identify what we want from our elected representatives;
- make informed and considered choices at the ballot box,
- hold our elected representatives accountable, including for promises made;
- denounce propaganda and political spin; and
- demand transparency.

If we don't demand good leadership, we have to accept bad leadership. The consequences of bad leadership can be potentially catastrophic for not only ourselves, but also for future generations. We need to make sure we do not fail them.

Exercise: Government Leadership

There are numerous views on the purpose of government:

- Government's role is to provide essential services; fulfill the fundamental duties of safety, prosperity, and justice; ensure the rights of each human; and protect the country so that its citizens, businesses, and organizations have the ability to pursue happiness, live a healthy life, and chase opportunities.

- Government's role is to introduce regulation and programs that balance economic growth, the distribution of resources, and the health, education, and fulfillment of citizens in different ways.

- Government's role is to reflect the public will.

- Governments are conservative institutions that create and sustain markets, enforcing systems of education and infrastructure that allow commerce to function effectively.

Consider the views listed above plus the traditional Aboriginal view of "caring for my place and all things in my place." Write down a sentence that reflects what you think the purpose of government is.

How informed are you on various government policies when you vote?

How well do you think our elected leaders are fulfilling their responsibilities?

What improvements do we need to demand from our elected leaders?

In accordance with Aboriginal spirituality, all of us—you . . . me . . . small business leaders . . . corporate leaders . . . and world leaders—have a responsibility to care for each other in the present, as well as a responsibility to provide for those who will follow us. In traditional times, our Elders always thought about the well-being of future generations they would never meet.

The world is in a state of imbalance. If we wait for world leaders to drive the changes needed to rectify the current state of this planet, that imbalance could remain for a very long time. Worse still, we could end up in a global state of disaster. We can't wait for world leaders to create a better world. We must be the leaders who do that. We need to somehow wed the economic/capitalist paradigm to the social/environmental imperative. A stepping stone of this courtship is in our own workplaces, where we can start conversations and nurture leadership that embraces environmental and social responsibility in partnership with profitability and fiscal prudence.

We all have a responsibility to lead. This could mean leading our life in a way that is true to who we are and to our life purpose. It could be leading a community group, a small business a cor poration, or a nation. Having been in senior leadership roles for more than twenty years, I know from experience how hard this can be. Being an introverted person, leadership was something I never aspired to, particularly after my breakdown. Whenever I carried out the duties of a particular role, my focus was always on doing the best job possible. I never thought about promotion or climbing the next rung on the corporate ladder. I didn't think I had the ability, and the thought of being a leader made my heart race with fear.

Each time I was asked to climb a rung, my immediate thought was to say no, but an inner voice always told me to say yes. After a period of time, it occurred to me that, spiritually, part of my Dreaming for whatever reason was to walk the footsteps of a leader. I begrudgingly realized that rather than fight my career path, I needed to embrace it and learn as much as I could so I could be the best leader I could be. I realized I needed to flow with the current and trust where life was taking me.

It was never easy. Being a leader is challenging both emotionally and intellectually. You must believe in both yourself and your personal journey to have the resilience needed to cope with the leadership roller coaster. If you don't, you leave the door open to self-doubt and anxiety.

Part of the leadership role is to ride external shocks that can occur at any time by remembering how to weather the storm (bend, be patient, learn, and grow). In my time, there have been many of these shocks:

- changes in policy;
- changes in budget;
- changes in staffing;
- changes in role;
- complaints from staff about each other;
- complaints from staff about me;
- being the subject of ongoing gossip;
- having to defend business decisions in the media (radio, television, and print);
- complaints from customers;
- political interference;

- ethical dilemmas;
- betrayal from those I trusted;
- racism; and
- unethical directives by people with greater influence than myself.

When I look back, although there have been instances that almost broke me, I can hold my head high knowing I always did my best and always treated those around me with respect.

This is my advice to anyone taking on a leadership role:

- Build your knowledge base.
- Believe in the role.
- Build a good team around you.
- Understand your role.
- Create a vision your team believes in.
- Delegate, empower, and provide the team with the skills and resources to get the job done.
- Build relationships.
- Communicate.
- Take on board advice but be prepared to make your own decisions.
- Be prepared to wear the consequences of your decisions.
- Learn from your mistakes.
- Remind yourself your job is what you do, not who you are.
- Be prepared to move on if you don't fit.

Ideally, when you are in a leadership role, there should be alignment between your personal values and those of the organization (for example, if you don't support gambling, you probably won't enjoy being a team leader at a casino). Compromising your inner self does not assist you in achieving well-being. If you are doing something you don't agree with, how hard is it going to be to tick the box for the second L, love? If you don't love what you are doing, it will be very hard for you to look, listen, learn, and lead. There have been two occasions in my career where it became very apparent that I was a square peg in a round hole and that to stay on would have been detrimental to myself and a variety of stakeholders. Moving on was heartbreaking but ultimately a good decision in both instances. Life isn't about jumping every hurdle you are given with stubborn resolve. Sometimes the best tactic is to walk around a hurdle.

If you are seeking leadership responsibilities because you need to feel important and powerful, then you are pursuing a leadership role for the wrong reason. Your driving force is not about love. It is underpinned by fear . . . fear of being seen as a failure . . . fear of not being important . . . fear of not feeling like you matter.

Before I had my breakdown, I was pursuing leadership responsibilities for the wrong reason. As my breakdown transformed into a breakthrough, I started to fulfill my leadership responsibilities for the right reason. This made it far easier for me to make the right decisions, to believe in myself, and to forgive myself when I made mistakes.

Are you comfortable with the leadership label or role? Many people are not. If so, how do you make the cloak of leadership a more comfortable garment to wear?

To be an effective leader, it is important to remember the importance of story. An effective leader understands:

- the organization's story (why the organization was created, its history, its current vision—its culture);
- the team's story (the team's role, how long it's been there, its influence, its connections, how effective it's been, the team dynamics and culture);
- the story of the leadership role you are in (how many leaders there have been, how the last leader was viewed); and
- the various individual team members' stories (who has been in the team the longest, who is new, who has influence, each person's motivation, and any external factors that might impact on their ability to get the job done).

If you are a leader, have you undertaken formal leadership training? Do you continuously review your leadership style and seek feedback on ways to improve? If there are opportunities for improvement (and there always are), you might need to undertake formal training and/or seek a coach or mentor.

In reviewing your leadership past, it is a good thing to identify your successes and what helped generate them (for example knowledge, confidence, collaboration, support, passion, belief). It is also good to review where things could have gone better, address any guilt issues, and think about what you have learned. In doing this, your leadership capabilities will continue to grow. Looking and listening are essential components of leadership; however, it is very important to analyze what you see and hear with the "filter" of truth. As an example, think about gossip. Gossip unfortunately goes with the territory of leadership. There will be gossip about you and there will be gossip about others. It is important you don't buy in to it.

Leadership involves teams. Teams are made up of people with unique skill sets, unique stories, and unique worldviews. Harnessing this diversity means extraordinary things can be achieved. This diversity can also create challenges relating to different team members' personal issues, anxieties, and doubts, which in turn can affect team harmony and productivity.

Creating the right workplace culture (including a focus on self-care) is important in getting the best out of each person as well as the best out of the team.

Leadership is about understanding story, having love and passion for what you do in life, listening to experts—people who have done it before you, people who can teach you. Then you will learn and one day you will become a leader. But you have got to lead by example.

A picture paints a thousand words and actions speak louder than words, so the message is clear: don't depend on words alone to achieve results. As a leader, it is important to say the right words and then back them up by showing the way with correct actions.

I was taught that before you make a decision, look beyond the decision and see what sort of effect it will have on the people you love. In traditional times, before Aboriginal people made a decision, they would look at how that decision would affect their tribe for generations to come and how it fitted in to the natural world and what effect it would have on that world.

So life was about thinking ahead for several generations

*and making positive decisions today that would benefit future
generations, not take away from future generations. So in
our world, the rivers would always stay clean, the trees would
always bear fruit, and nature in every way was taken care of
because we are a part of and belong to nature (Mother Earth).
My responsibility in life is to always pay respect to and care for
the land, my Mother, and to pass on the Lore of my people and
to walk that Lore in a humble way, hoping that other people will
follow.*

*When I was young, I was with an old man who was watching
television. On the screen were some politicians. As he watched
he started to become angry.*

*"See those fullas there, boy? They think they are leaders but
all they do is talk, talk, talk. They are nothing but ghosts. They
aren't leaving any tracks in the sand. Don't be a ghost: leave
some tracks for others to follow."*

*I have never forgotten what that old man said. If we don't
leave tracks then we haven't lived a good story. We must leave
tracks. We must lead in a way that is real.*

Think about your leadership or perhaps leaders you work under or even leaders you have seen on television.

Are there good tracks being left for others to follow or maybe
no tracks at all? Worse still, are the wrong tracks being left?

It is critical that we all aspire to be good leaders. It is also critical
that we demand good leadership from others. Good leadership:

- is flexible, strengths-based, and broader in scope than
  delivering results through others;

- embraces a holistic view of relationships, including connections that enhance community and environmental well-being;
- addresses disadvantage and supports equity;
- mitigates the likelihood of anthropogenic global catastrophe;
- embraces the six Ls (Lore, Love, Look, Listen, Learn, Lead);
- understands the importance of story;
- does things with the people, not for the people;
- makes decisions that take into consideration the impact on future generations;
- creates a better world;
- bends with the storm and learns from it;
- leads for the right reasons; and
- is authentic.

Navigating our way through life can be difficult. By creating, supporting, and nurturing outstanding leaders in government, corporations, companies, nongovernmental organizations, government organizations, and community organizations we will have a symphony of catalysts for positive change. As the world is renewed . . . as people are renewed . . . and as nature is renewed, balance will be restored and well-being easier to attain for all of us.

By doing this, we all have a greater chance to follow our Dreaming.

Message 30

True leadership includes caring for my place and all things in my place for my children's children's children's children.

Message 31

The world is off balance. Authentic, united leadership is our only hope for creating renewal and balance locally, nationally, and globally.

Message 32

Electing leaders is a privilege we must respect, honor, and carry out with due diligence.

Message 33

Don't wait for world leaders to create a better world. You be the leader for a better world.

Message 34

Lead for the right reasons.

Message 35

Don't be a ghost. Leave some tracks for others to follow.

Epilogue

The Old People say, "When we leave this world behind, all we leave behind is our story, so make it the best story possible."

We are conceived in love and born in love to achieve this purpose. The Dreaming Path tells us our story should be framed by a commitment to caring for our place and all things in our place.

This doesn't mean we don't have freedom in how we do that. In fact, it is the exact opposite: we are all unique, as are our footsteps and our story. It is up to us to embrace that uniqueness, to dance with diversity and have the courage to be different.

Through providing you with an understanding of the Lore, we hope to give you a new way to view the world and your part in it. We hope this book and the thoughts we have shared help you reflect on your journey and where it is heading. Much of our thought is captured in these messages:

- Care for your place and all things in your place.
- Everything and everyone has a story. The more stories we share, the more we learn. The more we learn, the more we

grow. The more we grow, the closer we are to achieving well-being—individually and universally.

- It is vital for each of us to create, nurture, and sustain relationships, including with the land, babies, children, young people, young adults, adults, parents, Elders, and the very old.
- Our celebration of diversity must be underpinned by a platform of unity.
- Always share.
- We are conceived in love, born into love, and surrounded by love. The love of the Mother, Father, and Spirit Ancestors is always there for us.
- Carry out loving deeds for others and yourself as often as you can.
- Give thanks every day for the abundance of good things that surround you.
- Be humble in all you do.
- Look, listen, and learn. The world that surrounds you is your classroom.
- If you come to me knowing everything, I can teach you nothing. If you come to me knowing nothing, I can teach you everything.
- Knowledge is worth nothing if we don't share it.
- Seek truth in all that you do.
- Your life's journey has a purpose. It is special and individual—just like you. Respect it, honor it, own it, and walk it.
- Every day is an opportunity to be inspired and to inspire others.

- Feeling empowered requires you to believe in yourself and your journey. As you shine, don't let others dim your light: they can't if you don't let them.
- When the storms of life appear, face them with faith in what you have learned and what you will learn. Bend; don't break.
- Each time you overcome hardship, recognize and celebrate your courage and resilience.
- Your past is an important path to your present. Acknowledge, accept, and learn from your past and address those things that are preventing you from finding contentment in the now.
- Too much focus on the future distracts you from the magic of the present.
- Embrace change.
- Laugh often.
- When loss occurs, allow yourself to grieve and heal.
- Your Dreaming is about your life and what you do with it. Part of your Dreaming is to connect to the Dreaming Path.
- View the world from beyond the Western perspective. By learning from other cultures, you will live a more fulfilling story and help create a better world.
- To care for others, we need to first care for ourselves.
- We need to flow like water. We reach our destination by calmly accepting the twists and turns ahead of us and adjusting our course as we see fit, meandering in synchronicity with what is around us.
- Living a good story means no one gets left behind.
- Don't give your power away to the chatter of your mind.

- True leadership includes caring for my place and all things in my place for my children's children's children's children.
- The world is off balance. Authentic, united leadership is our only hope for creating renewal and balance locally, nationally, and globally.
- Electing leaders is a privilege we must respect, honor, and carry out with due diligence.
- Don't wait for world leaders to create a better world. You be the leader for a better world.
- Lead for the right reasons.
- Don't be a ghost. Leave some tracks for others to follow.

Many of us are not living the best story possible. We are not living our truth. This undermines our well-being and the well-being of our communities, nations, and the world itself.

The world is in crisis and closer to human-made global catastrophe than it ever has been. The planet is overheating as Country burns and ice caps melt. A pandemic invades all countries on earth, striking down the old and vulnerable with impassive efficiency. Protests erupt across the globe as those forced to the margins of society say "no more" to corruption, environmental destruction, inequality, and racism—but are our leaders listening?

We, the current custodians of this planet, have a responsibility to change what has gone wrong.

It is time for us to unite and be clear in our purpose. It is time for renewal.

Global renewal starts with personal renewal. It is up to each of us to understand how special we are . . . to take ownership of our lives . . . to walk our footsteps and live our truth. This is the path to contentment, inner peace, and well-being each of us can create if we are humble enough to look, listen, and learn, and then courageous enough to take action. The Dreaming Path and the Lore can guide us to this path.

Before we act, we need to address any scars from the past that are affecting our ability to fully embrace the present. Individually, collectively, and globally, we need to heal.

Healing myself after my breakdown was the hardest thing I have ever done. It was also the best thing I have ever done. My healing journey started as a process of renewal that turned into a process of transformation. By finding my true self, I was able to like myself for the first time. I learned to see myself through the eyes of the Father and the Mother and the Spirit Ancestors and understand that I am never alone and also that I am worthy of the love that surrounds us all. This has enabled me to walk Country and feel the magic that surrounds me. To dance with the trees, to dance with the wind, to dance with spirit. From a place of devastating loss, I have been able to live a story of profound gratitude.

My hope is that, through the insights Uncle Paul and I have shared, you can dance with what is around you in your own unique way as well, and also live a story you never dreamed possible.

Uncle Paul and I have to leave the fireside for a little while . . . but these flames . . . flames of love . . . flames of hope . . . and flames of unity will continue to burn. They will be here for us when we return and sit down once again.

Until then, Uncle Paul and I wish you well on your journey.

May you enjoy the sunshine and be bathed by the golden glow of the moon as you experience the magic of nature and what surrounds you each day.

May your Dreaming be a strong one and your story the best story possible.

Acknowledgments

I give thanks to the earth, our Mother, for all she and her children give us.

This book wouldn't have been possible had I not met Uncle Paul Gordon so many years ago. To Uncle Paul, I give thanks for the knowledge he has shared, for the learning he has catalyzed, and for being a good friend. In many ways, I have written this book as a means of introducing him to a world that can benefit so much from his wisdom.

In the same breath, I acknowledge Peter McDonough, an outstanding role model for me. Peter, your humility and passion, and your gentle but uncompromising commitment to Aboriginal culture and ways of being, are inspiring.

To my wife, Alison, I say the biggest thank you. You told your family you were going to marry me the day after we met. You brought our three beautiful children into the world and taught me about kindness and love. You stood by me through my breakdown despite some saying you should run. You supported me when I started my cultural journey and embraced the learning I shared within our family. Your faith in our future didn't waver when I left my executive role in government and started my own business, and your enthusiasm for my desire to write about our culture has always been off the charts. With the publishing of *The Dreaming Path*, I can now say, "Alison, we did it!"

To our children, Rhys, Brianna, and Liam, thank you for your continued expressions of love and telling me I am the best dad ever. Although the criteria you use for this assessment might be a bit dodgy, being your dad is the greatest blessing I could ever have wished for.

Friends come and go, but not Kieran and Sharon Quigley. I give my thanks for more than forty years of friendship and your enthusiasm, excitement, and interest in my writing journey. As non-Aboriginal people, you had no understanding of Aboriginal culture and spirituality to start with, and yet you were open to listening and learning. Your belief in my dream gives me hope.

The creation of *The Dreaming Path* started with a phone conversation with a man named Gregory Messina, an American literary agent living in Paris, about promoting a book that would draw on Australian Aboriginal culture and spirituality. Go figure! Greg, thank you for embracing me so quickly and connecting me to the wonderful people at HarperOne.

HarperOne have been such a wonderful team in preparing this book for US readers. In particular, I extend the biggest thank you to Gabi Page-Fort who has been an inspiration to me. Her passion and belief in the messages I wish to share gives me hope for a better world where each of us can live the best story possible.

To those I have been out bush with, who I have danced with, who I have shared ceremony with, who I have shared stories with, I would like to thank you for being part of my life story.

About the Authors

Paul Callaghan is an Aboriginal man belonging to the land of the Worimi people, located on the coast of New South Wales just north of Newcastle.

For many years he has held senior executive positions in Aboriginal- and non-Aboriginal-related service areas, but eventually his desire to focus on community and individual well-being compelled him to start his own business. *The Dreaming Path* was awarded the 2023 Australian Industry Awards Small Publishers' Adult Book of the Year "for deftly publishing culturally sensitive and protected material to a mass market."

In addition to consultancy work, Paul is a motivational speaker, a storyteller, a dancer, and an author. In 2019 his manuscript of a novel titled *Coincidence* was short-listed for the inaugural Daisy Utemorrah Award. The short-listing inspired Paul to undertake and complete a PhD in Creative Practice, which included the creation of a novel titled *Consequence*. In June 2023, *The Dreaming Path* was announced the Australian Book Industry Awards Small Publishers' Book of the Year.

Paul's passions are driven by his belief in the power of story to create a better world.

Uncle Paul Gordon is a Ngemba man, born at Brewarrina in the land now called Australia. He grew up in a tin hut on the Barwon River in northwestern New South Wales (NSW). Since 1983, he has spent most of his time with the Old Men performing cultural activities and learning Aboriginal Lore. Today, Uncle Paul is recognized as a senior Elder, and he is one of the highest initiated Aboriginal men in NSW. He contributed many of the stories in *The Dreaming Path*.

About the Cover Artwork

Our Lore encompasses everything. Everything we know and don't know must sit within the Lore, which is represented by circles within circles. Every circle represents learning and lessons to understand in the physical world and in the spiritual world. Wawaii (the rainbow serpent/s) is shown in the colors of the rainbow. Where he/she has traveled, he/she has created waterholes in Mother Earth that never go dry. They are everywhere.

There are other circles in the painting that represent more Lore, and also represent waterholes and/or family groups.

You will see emu and kangaroo footprints. This shows that both men and women have a responsibility to the Lore and they walk together. The image is shown on rock to show my respect for my cultural grandfather's (Paul Gordon's) people.

Water flows over the Country, providing life for all.